Essential Guide to Educational Supervision in Postgraduate Medical Education

Essential Guide to Educational Supervision in Postgraduate Medical Education

EDITED BY

NICOLA COOPER MRCP

Consultant in Acute Medicine and Geriatrics
The Leeds Teaching Hospitals NHS Trust
Leeds, UK

KIRSTY FORREST MMEd FRCA

Consultant in Anaesthesia and Education
The Leeds Teaching Hospitals NHS Trust
Leeds, UK

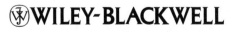

WILEY-BLACKWELL

A John Wiley & Sons, Ltd., Publication

BMJ|Books

This edition first published 2009, © 2009 by Blackwell Publishing Ltd

BMJ Books is an imprint of BMJ Publishing Group Limited, used under licence by Blackwell Publishing which was acquired by John Wiley & Sons in February 2007. Blackwell's publishing programme has been merged with Wiley's global Scientific, Technical and Medical business to form Wiley-Blackwell.

Registered office: John Wiley & Sons Ltd, The Atrium, Southern Gate, Chichester, West Sussex, PO19 8SQ, UK

Editorial offices: 9600 Garsington Road, Oxford, OX4 2DQ, UK
                       The Atrium, Southern Gate, Chichester, West Sussex, PO19 8SQ, UK
                       111 River Street, Hoboken, NJ 07030-5774, USA

For details of our global editorial offices, for customer services and for information about how to apply for permission to reuse the copyright material in this book please see our website at www.wiley.com/wiley-blackwell

Library of Congress Cataloging-in-Publication Data

Essential guide to educational supervision in postgraduate medical education / edited by
Nicola Cooper, Kirsty Forrest.
      p. ; cm.
   Includes bibliographical references.
   ISBN 978-1-4051-7071-0
   1. Medicine—Study and teaching (Continuing education)—Great Britain. 2. Mentoring in
medicine—Great Britain. I. Cooper, Nicola. II. Forrest, Kirsty.
   [DNLM: 1. Education, Medical, Continuing—organization & administration—Great Britain.
2. Education, Medical, Graduate—organization & administration—Great Britain. 3. Clinical Competence—
Great Britain. 4. Mentors—education—Great Britain. 5. Teaching—methods—Great Britain. 6. Vocational
Guidance—Great Britain. W20 E78 2009]
   R845.E77 2009
   610.71'141—dc22   2008039508

ISBN: 978-1-4051-7071-0

A catalogue record for this book is available from the British Library.

Set in 9.5/12 Meridien by Macmillan Publishing Solutions, Chennai, India
(www.macmillansolutions.com)
Printed and bound in the United Kingdom by TJ International Ltd, Padstow, Cornwall

3   2010

Contents

List of Contributors

Julian Archer MBChB, MRCPCH, PhD
Clinical Lecturer in Medical Education, Peninsula College of Medicine and Dentistry
Associate Director of Research, Healthcare Assessment and Training (HCAT), Plymouth, UK

Jonathan Beard ChM, MEd, FRCS
Foundation Training Programme Director, Sheffield Teaching Hospitals
Honorary Professor of Surgical Education, University of Sheffield, Sheffield, UK

Peter Belfield BSc MBChB FRCP
Consultant Geriatrician and Educational Supervisor
Deputy Medical Director, Joint Royal Colleges of Physicians Training Board and The Leeds Teaching Hospitals (Professional Development and Education) Leeds, UK

David Clegg BA(Hons), DipCG, PDGCCI
Senior Careers Consultant, University of Leeds
Regional Careers Manager, Yorkshire Deanery, Leeds, UK

Nicola Cooper MRCP
Consultant in Acute Medicine and Geriatrics, The Leeds Teaching Hospitals NHS Trust, Leeds, UK

Carolyn S. Evans FRCA
Consultant Anaesthetist, Bradford Teaching Hospitals NHS Foundation Trust
Regional Adviser for Anaesthesia, Yorkshire and the Humber Postgraduate Deanery, Bradford, UK

Kathy Feest PhD, BA(Hons), Cert Med Ed
Associate Dean and Director of Foundation School, Severn Deanery
Special Advisor to Foundation Programme, UK Foundation Programme Office, Bristol, UK

Kirsty Forrest MMEd FRCA
Consultant in Anaesthesia and Education, The Leeds Teaching Hospitals NHS Trust, Leeds, UK

Jane V. Howard MBBS, FRCA
Consultant in Anaesthesia and Intensive Care Medicine, Leeds General Infirmary
Foundation Training Programme Director, Foundation Year 2, The West Yorkshire Foundation School, Leeds, UK

Alastair McGowan OBE, FRCP, FRCS, FRCA, FCEM
Dean of Postgraduate Medicine
  for the West of Scotland, NHS
  Education for Scotland,
  Glasgow, UK

Judy McKimm MBA, MA(Ed), BA(Hons), Cert Ed, FHEA
Senior Lecturer, Centre for Medical
  and Healthcare Sciences, University
  of Auckland, New Zealand
Visiting Professor of Healthcare
  Education and Leadership,
  University of Bedfordshire,
  Luton, UK

Colin R. Melville MBChB, FRCA, FRCP(Glasg)
Foundation School Director,
  North Yorkshire East Coast
  Foundation School
Honorary Senior Clinical Lecturer,
  Hull York Medical School

Consultant in Emergency and
  Intensive Care Medicine, Hull
  and East Yorkshire NHS Trust,
  Hull, UK

Rosalind Roden DRCOG, DCH, Dip IMC, FRCS, FCEM
Associate Postgraduate Dean for
  Careers and Personal Development,
  Yorkshire and the Humber
  Postgraduate Deanery Chair,
  ATLS® Steering Group, The Royal
  College of Surgeons of England,
  London, UK

Sean Smith MSc, MBCS
Webmaster, The Yorkshire Deanery,
University of Leeds, Leeds, UK

Sean Williamson MBChB, FRCA
Consultant Anaesthetist, The
James Cook University Hospital,
Middlesbrough, UK

Foreword

The editors have developed an excellent book which brings together a wide range of practical advice from national and international experts, who have a wealth of experience of training junior doctors.

Educational supervision has always been important, but as we enter the next decade it will be even more vital to ensure well trained and supported doctors progress through training. The European Working Time Directive, changes in hospital practice such as shorter length of stay, the shift to community working, and less contact with clinical supervisors all make the mentorship and facilitated, valuable learning offered by a good educational supervisor of critical significance. There is a move away from educational supervision being an 'add on' for busy consultants to a clear role that is planned, protected and valued. Hospital doctors have much to learn from training in general practice where such valuable time is more ring fenced. Increasingly, educational supervisors will be professionally selected, trained and paid for their work. They will also be held to account for standards of practice as defined by the Postgraduate Medical Education and Training Board (PMETB), as education and training are ever more quality assured.

This book should become essential reading for all those involved in education and training. There are superb sections on the whole range of educational activities which a successful educational supervisor will encounter, from how to deal with e-portfolios to the particularly challenging area of doctors in difficulty. There is something here for everyone and the chapters on learning and reflection are something we as trainers can all utilise ourselves. The Appendices usefully finish the book, with a number of example scenarios which bring to life some of the challenges faced in becoming a good supervisor. All the chapters help you develop your trainees more effectively. The Editors have ensured high quality contributions which make this a key addition to the literature in this field.

Training systems, regulatory bodies and guidance for trainers may change regularly, but excellent educational supervision will always help trainees throughout their postgraduate education, which in turn will improve the quality of care for patients for years to come.

Peter Belfield BSc MBChB FRCP
February 2009

Acknowledgements

There are many people to thank for their help with this book: the expert authors who gave of their time generously, and were great at keeping to deadlines; Mary Banks from Wiley-Blackwell who suggested the need for such a book and made it possible; and Alison Lansbury and Richard Fuller for their helpful suggestions and advice.

On a more personal note, we would like to thank our families and friends for their love and support during the process.

Last but not least, thanks also to all the fantastic trainees we have worked with, who we always kept in mind during the development of this book and who make it a real pleasure to be an educational supervisor.

Nicola Cooper and Kirsty Forrest

Introduction

Consultants and general practitioners spend years learning to be clinical specialists. Yet their role often requires them to supervise the education and training of other doctors. Many of those who want to do this job well feel unprepared for the task.

Questions and concerns keep arising in the minds of colleagues who are educational supervisors. We hope to answer these questions in this book, and have deliberately tried to keep things practical as well as describe some of the theory that underpins recommended practice.

What is an educational supervisor?

Different documents describe the roles and responsibilities of an educational supervisor, which are outlined in Boxes 1–3. To fulfil all these requirements and possess all of these attributes could be considered quite challenging! However, the simpler 'job plan' described by Carolyn S. Evans in Chapter 1 is definitely more palatable. Dr Evans divides the post into three parts with pastoral, educational and administrative components; the chapters that follow are also broadly divided this way.

These components reflect the process of educational supervision: building a relationship, ensuring that learning takes place and monitoring and appraising the whole process. Chapter 1 gives an overview of the educational supervisor's responsibilities, many of which are then developed in further chapters.

Box 1

The Association for Medical Education in Europe (AMEE) produced a guide entitled 'Effective educational and clinical supervision' [1], which was based on a literature review and a questionnaire survey. The authors define educational supervision as, 'the provision of guidance and feedback on matters of personal, professional and educational development in the context of a trainee's experience of providing safe and appropriate patient care.' The key points highlighted in this guide are as follows.
- Effective supervision should be in context, that is, the supervisor should know the requirements of the training body.

(Continued)

> **Box 1** (Continued)
>
> - Direct supervision (when the supervisor and trainee work together and observe each other) has a positive impact on patient outcome and trainee development.
> - Frequent constructive feedback is essential.
> - Supervision should be structured with regular meetings.
> - Supervision should include clinical matters, teaching and research, management/administration, pastoral care, interpersonal skills, personal development and reflection.
> - The quality of the supervisory relationship strongly affects the effectiveness of supervision.
> - Supervisors need training in medical education, counselling skills, assessment, appraisal, feedback, careers advice and interpersonal skills.
> - Supervisors need to understand helpful supervisory behaviours and ineffective supervisory behaviours.

What relationship do I have with the trainee?

The topic of personal support does not cause as much concern as the topic of 'how to deal with doctors in difficulty'. However, if you get personal support right you may not have an escalating problem on your hands. Many of us believe that we know how to be personable and a good listener. However, this is not the same as offering support, challenging behaviours and developing learning.

Judy McKimm lays out the process of guidance and support, which includes being explicit about roles and having very clear ground rules that can stop you and the trainee from getting confused. In Appendix 1, Dr McKimm also provides helpful scenarios to accompany the chapter.

How do I deal with a problem trainee?

Doctors in difficulty can take a disproportionate amount of an educational supervisor's time. In Chapter 3, Rosalind Roden, with 10 years experience at the Deanery level in this area, explains the various reasons why a doctor can get into difficulties and what to do about it.

As always, the simplest instructions are the best – gather as much information as you can and write everything down, a lesson usually personally learned the hard way. This chapter is also helpful for one's own health and you may be able to spot if your see-saw is out of kilter. Again in Appendix 1, example scenarios are provided by Dr Roden to help the reader work through real but anonymous examples of common problems.

Box 2

The different requirements of an educational supervisor
The GMC lists a set of professional and then personal attributes of a
doctor with responsibilities for educational supervision [2]. The personal
attributes are:
- enthusiasm for his/her specialty;
- a personal commitment to teaching and learning;
- sensitivity and responsiveness to the educational needs of students
  and junior doctors;
- the capacity to promote development of the required professional
  attitudes and values;
- an understanding of the principles of education as applied to
  medicine;
- an understanding of research method;
- practical teaching skills;
- a willingness to develop both as a doctor and as a teacher;
- a commitment to audit and peer review of his/her teaching;
- the ability to use formative assessment (e.g. work-based assessments)
  for the benefit of the student/trainee and
- the ability to carry out formal appraisals.

How can I be useful to a trainee's career?

Careers advice and guidance is often sought by trainees from their supervisors. However, research suggests that this is poorly given. Chapter 4 has
been jointly written by a clinician and a professional careers advisor. It sets
out how to approach both individual and group guidance with many practical tips for educational supervisors. Helping a trainee to find the most appropriate specialty for his abilities and skills must be one of the most rewarding
aspects of a supervisor's role.

I have to organise a training programme, where do I start?

While it is not essential to have a qualification in medical education to be
an educational supervisor, it does help. The 'Gold Guide' (Box 3) states
that educational supervisors should 'have an understanding of educational
theory'.

Sometimes, what is lacking is a grasp of the 'bigger picture' when it
comes to education, so Chapter 5 gives an overview of what a curriculum
involves and how to put one into practice, with some food for thought and
examples.

> **Box 3**
>
> According to the 'Gold Guide', a guide to postgraduate specialty training in the UK, educational supervisors should [3]:
>
> - be adequately prepared for the role and have an understanding of educational theory and practical educational techniques, for example have undertaken formal facilitated training or an online training programme or participate in relevant training-the-trainers programmes;
> - be trained to offer educational supervision and undertake appraisal and feedback;
> - undertake training in competence assessment for specialty training;
> - be trained in equality and diversity;
> - provide regular appraisal opportunities, which should take place at the beginning, middle and end of a placement;
> - develop a learning agreement and educational objectives with the trainee, which is mutually agreed and is the point of reference for future appraisal;
> - be responsible for ensuring that trainees whom they supervise maintain and develop their specialty learning portfolio and participate in the specialty assessment process;
> - provide regular feedback to the trainee on their progress;
> - ensure that the structured report, which is a detailed review and synopsis of the trainee's learning portfolio, is returned within the necessary timescales;
> - contact the employer (usually the medical director) and the postgraduate dean in case the level of performance of a trainee is of concern;
> - be able to advise the trainee about access to career management;
> - be responsible for their educational role to the training programme director and locally to the employer's lead for postgraduate medical education.

How can I help trainees learn?

Educational supervisors are in the business of professional education, which is broader than training, and developing professional expertise, which is more than competence. In Chapter 6, some principles of professional education are discussed, followed by some tips on how to 'teach' excellence, and then an overview of learning styles.

Written by two educationalists, the teaching and learning chapter is a whirlwind tour of some key concepts in postgraduate medical education that educational supervisors need to know about.

Reflective portfolios – why?

Reflection in postgraduate medical education is often misunderstood, yet it can be an intellectually rigorous process. It is an important and evidence-based component in the development of expertise. Good trainees reflect all the time, and reflection is discussed in the teaching and learning chapter. In Chapter 7, Kathy Feest discusses narrative reflection, its origins and purpose. Narrative reflection is just one way of reflecting. Narratives are a way of 'formalising' how we know we already learn, that is through stories, and can be powerful learning tools.

Reflective practice, of course, also applies to educational supervisors as well as to trainees. The task set at the end of this chapter is a challenging one that we hope you will engage in.

Assessments – why so many of them, what's the evidence?

Have you ever wondered why 360-degree feedback is valid even when trainees can choose their own assessors? Or what the purposes of work-based assessments are? Or how they contribute to assessing a trainee's overall performance? Or what the difference between assessment and appraisal is?

Julian Archer gives an overview of the science behind the current work-based assessments in postgraduate medical education. Chapter 8 explains some key concepts in assessment generally, their purpose in postgraduate medical education, the importance of assessor training and the ways to judge a trainee's performance. The important matter of feedback is discussed in some detail, as this is an action that is often performed poorly, yet is vital if work-based assessments are to be educationally effective.

E-portfolio ... I'm rubbish with computers!

Unfortunately for some, there is no way of doing the job of an educational supervisor without using information technology (IT). Many supervisors are 'digital immigrants' as opposed to their younger trainees who are 'digital natives'.

Sean Smith explains some of the terminology used, and the role of IT in postgraduate medical education, including Web 2.0 and wikis.

How do I know I'm doing a good job?

Being reviewed by the Postgraduate Medical Education and Training Board (PMETB) can be a daunting prospect, but Chapter 10 provides an overview of what quality assurance means in practice.

Many educational supervisors are enthusiastic and committed to their own personal development (reading this book is an example!) but for those who also organise training programmes, an understanding of the bigger picture in terms of quality assurance is vital.

Post script

Appendix 1 at the end of this book gives an historical overview and outlines the current proposed structure for postgraduate medical training in the UK.

Although the word 'trainee' is used to talk about doctors who have not completed their formal postgraduate education, this is an unsatisfactory term. Training, from an educational point of view, implies a person who is learning to adequately perform a task, whereas education is something more than that, particularly professional education. The word 'trainee' also implies that those who have completed their formal training no longer need to learn.

However, trainee is a commonly used term and, in the absence of a better word, we use it in this book to mean a doctor who is on a formal postgraduate programme and who has not yet obtained a 'certificate of completion of training' (CCT).

We realise that we may not have answered everyone's questions when it comes to being an educational supervisor – in fact, we may have generated more questions than answers in some cases! This is why we have added further resources, where appropriate, for you to explore subjects in more detail. We hope you get as much out of reading this book as we did in editing it!

Nicola Cooper and Kirsty Forrest

July 2008

References

1. Kilminster S, Cottrel D, Grant J, Jolly B. AMEE Guide no. 27: effective educational and clinical supervision. *Med Teach* 2007; **29**: 2–19.
2. General Medical Council. The doctor as teacher. GMC, London, 1999.
3. A guide to postgraduate specialty training in the UK (The gold guide) (2007) URL http://www.mmc.nhs.uk/default.aspx?page=315

CHAPTER 1

How to be an educational supervisor

Carolyn S. Evans
Bradford Teaching Hospitals NHS Foundation Trust; Yorkshire and the Humber
Postgraduate Deanery, UK

The educational supervisor is not a new concept – it was established in 1987 – but the role has become far more prominent following the implementation of Modernising Medical Careers (MMC), which introduced shorter, more focussed, competency-based postgraduate training programmes. The importance of the role of educational supervisor is emphasised in the General Medical Council (GMC) publication 'The New Doctor' [1], produced in conjunction with the Postgraduate Medical Education and Training Board (PMETB). This focuses on the generic standards for training within the foundation years, a period of critical transition from medical student to doctor in which the educational supervisor can be pivotal in ensuring trainee survival and enjoyment as well as advising on career pathways. Equally difficult demands are made of educational supervisors responsible for trainees appointed to core training (CT) and specialty training (ST) posts in run-through training programmes, as well as those advising trainees in fixed-term specialty training appointments (FTSTA) after August 2007. The importance and relevance of educational supervision is enshrined in all specialty-specific competency-based curricula; for example, the Royal College of Anaesthetists states that every trainee must have an educational supervisor.

Educational supervision is not just about the educational aspects of postgraduate medical education; and if you are thinking this is not relevant, just ask yourself the following questions:

- Who took an interest in my welfare?
- Who helped uncover my hidden talent?
- Who has been a useful role model for me?
- Who helped me face and resolve a difficult situation in my personal or professional life?
- Who helped me acquire new vision or direction?

Essential Guide to Educational Supervision in Postgraduate Medical Education.
Edited by Nicola Cooper and Kirsty Forrest. © 2009 Blackwell Publishing,
ISBN: 978-1-4051-7071-0.

Supervision

Supervision is a term that can lead to different interpretations. It does not mean someone looking over your shoulder all the time! Educational supervision incorporates both hierarchical and evaluative concepts and can be seen as having supportive, educational and administrative functions.

Under the umbrella of educational supervision, *clinical* supervision has been defined as 'an exchange between practicing professionals to enable the development of professional skills' [2]. The individuals involved are usually in different stages of training and these exchanges form an essential part of the journey from novice to expert.

Supervision in the clinical environment includes a clear demarcation of who is reporting to whom. This may involve a formal process or consist of an informal discussion over coffee. We all undertake clinical supervision to a greater or lesser extent during our normal working day in any situation where we come into contact with someone less experienced than ourselves. This provides part of the information gathered by the educational supervisor for discussion with the trainee. The educational supervisor takes the views of clinical supervisors and uses these to inform the support, development and assessment of the trainee's performance.

Educational supervision may at times expand to take on a mentoring role in which a guidance and developmental conversation leads to a more wide-ranging discussion. In this context, the topics discussed should remain confidential unless permission to disclose them is given by the trainee.

The purpose of educational supervision

Educational supervisors are gatekeepers whose role is to maintain standards of training to all levels of trainees in all specialities. To achieve this, the educational supervisors must understand the educational objectives of each period of training for which they have responsibility. They should ensure priority is given to the educational component of the post and that the trainee is not overloaded with inappropriate responsibilities or excessive clinical commitments. An effective educational supervisor should contribute to the development of professionalism and self-confidence in the trainee and to the reduction of work-related stress, especially for those in their initial years of training.

Becoming an educational supervisor

There is no formal job description for an educational supervisor although the Faculty of Occupational Medicine does specify that educational supervisors must be on the GMC's specialist register and be approved by their local specialist training committee [3]. The essential requirements are an interest in trainee education and development, an understanding of the appropriate programmes, and readiness to commit time beyond that formally allocated as supporting professional activity (SPA) within the consultant job plan.

An individual does not need to have responsibility for training within a department in order to take on the role of educational supervisor. In small departments with less than 10 trainees it may be possible for the college tutor to act as educational supervisor for all the trainees but normal practice is for the educational supervisor to be an additional rung on the educational ladder, accountable to the college tutor. The Royal College of Anaesthetists' view is that educational supervisors should be career grade doctors, for example consultants, staff grades or associate specialists. Senior trainees, as part of their professional development, may be offered the opportunity to take on a supervisory role for a junior trainee but will require appropriate support and regular review by the college tutor [4].

In some specialties, educational supervisors are allocated to trainees by the training programme director or college tutor, which ensures that all trainees have an identified educational supervisor at the start of their post. However, the opportunity to change educational supervisor must be available should the partnership not prove constructive. Although practice varies between trusts, the trainee usually keeps the same educational supervisor for the duration of their attachment in that hospital.

Some deaneries offer generic training programmes for educational supervisors, which cover assessments in competency-based training programmes, appraisal skills, career guidance, teaching skills and mentoring, all facets of effective educational supervision. There is concern that there is no standard education or supervisory skills course available and that the majority of educational supervisors have had no formal educational training. The Mersey Deanery, reviewing the contribution of educational supervisors in the foundation years, found that 51% had not received any formal training [5].

It is essential for the educational supervisor to understand the educational objectives of the specific period of training for which he or she has responsibility. Trainees interviewed in their second-year foundation programme felt the recent changes in postgraduate medical training had left their educational supervisors unclear of what was required of an F2 trainee [6]. Neither trainee nor supervisor will benefit if both are working in the dark with no clear idea of where they are going.

Key skills of an educational supervisor include the ability to:
- Teach;
- Facilitate rather than direct;
- Challenge without being threatening;
- Provide career guidance and
- Mentor.

Educational supervisors fail in their role for a variety of reasons. This may be because they are rigid in their approach, they always offer minimal support or empathy, they are not interested in teaching or they are unable to encourage or praise and always highlight the trainee's deficiencies. One or more of these may apply when a person does not enjoy the responsibility and challenges of being an educational supervisor but it is not necessary to exhibit all of these to get excused.

If the educational supervisor cannot engage with the trainee in a constructive manner, the training programme director or college tutor should be contacted as soon as possible to resolve the issue. It may be necessary to allocate an alternative supervisor. Educational supervisors should be allocated without any bias in ethnicity, sexual orientation or gender of the individuals concerned, but occasionally serious differences of opinion or personality clashes will occur. An open admission of a failing supervisory relationship is more constructive than leaving the trainee to flounder and get nowhere.

Educational supervisor responsibilities

Meeting and appraisals

The first meeting is very important and time should be set aside for this in a private office. The objectives of the meeting are to agree on the purpose and role of the relationship, to establish an understanding with the trainee and to agree future means of communication. The trainee should leave the meeting feeling supported and clear about expectations. The most sensible and well-established structure is to agree on a personal development plan (PDP) with some short- and long-term educational goals. The educational supervisor should establish a timetable for future meetings to review progress and respond to any underperformance.

The trainee's PDP should be amended and updated at each meeting. Effective feedback is an important component of these discussions and is aimed at raising confidence and motivating the trainee. The educational supervisor should confirm areas of strength and areas for development. These may relate to lack of clinical exposure, specific clinical skills or broader issues such as communication. Targets must be set and agreed, and both parties should sign a record of the meeting. If the trainee is keeping a log book of cases or procedures undertaken as part of a training portfolio, a regular review by the educational supervisor can be a positive start to a meeting. The data reviewed can also direct the trainee's PDP targets for the next few months.

Guidance on postgraduate examinations

Examinations are an inevitable part of the educational supervisory discussion because in many specialties progress depends on passing royal college examinations by a certain point within the programme. The educational supervisor should know about local examination courses and the study leave budget, and be able to offer advice on appropriate regional and national revision courses for the failing trainee. If educational supervisors know their trainees well, they can direct them to the relevant support (Box 1.1).

Box 1.1

A trainee with appropriate knowledge but who continued to fail despite attending examination preparation courses was offered the opportunity of being video-assessed in order to analyse her presentation skills. This bought about a dramatic change in her body language and delivery in the oral examination and she passed the next sitting of the examination effortlessly. Her educational supervisor organised this session at the deanery with input from an educationalist and was able to maximise the use of this resource by knowing the trainee and her weaknesses.

Educational supervisors should also get involved in the local institution's examination preparation programme, for example teaching sessions, local courses and mock examinations.

There are huge personal and professional implications when a trainee keeps failing postgraduate examinations. It is a very public display of failure to progress. Educational supervisors will be aware of the pressure that working for examinations produces in such individuals. Putting time limits on essential educational targets increases the pressure on the trainee.

Educational supervisors need to know how many attempts trainees can have and what happens if they persistently fail an examination. Some colleges offer guidance interviews for failing trainees; the educational supervisor is the ideal person to accompany the trainee to these meetings, both for support and to ensure that suggestions from the panel are implemented. The Royal College of Anaesthetists report that if trainees attend a guidance interview alone they may feel unable to ask questions of the panel and may later have very limited recollection of the advice offered.

When a trainee is persistently failing postgraduate examinations it may fall to the educational supervisor to start the process of exploring other career options. This can be difficult, especially if the trainee has no insight into the reasons for his or her failure to progress; taking another colleague along to reinforce the message can be helpful.

Career advice

Predictions of staffing requirements in all specialties continue to be difficult, but an educational supervisor should have a feel for employment prospects now and in the future, especially in order to advise foundation programme trainees about CT posts versus run-through training programmes. Those in CT posts will need guidance when applying for entry to an ST programme, including reviewing their application form, giving realistic advice on the likelihood of success, advising them where to apply and ensuring they are considering other employment options if the ST programmes are extremely competitive.

Interview practice is valued and appreciated by all trainees regardless of the level of post being sought.

Although educational supervisors are unlikely to be experts on the constantly changing guidance on 'less than full-time training' (flexible training), they should know where to direct trainees for advice. Each deanery will have an identified person with responsibility for flexible training. The trainee will also need to meet with a specialty-specific advisor to explore details of how flexible training can be incorporated into a training programme. Although the majority of requests for flexible training are related to domestic commitments, it may be appropriate for an educational supervisor to suggest becoming a flexible trainee for a period of time if an individual's health precludes working full-time, such as a trainee with poorly controlled diabetes, an acute depressive illness or a recurrence of a chronic problem such as Crohn's disease or multiple sclerosis.

Arranging access to flexible training can enable a trainee to return to work much sooner than would otherwise be possible, although trainees must be working at least 50% of full-time hours, including on-call work, for their time to be counted towards a Certificate of Completion of Training (CCT). Educational supervisors play an essential role in enabling this type of flexible work and then monitoring and supporting the trainee once it has been established.

Locum doctors could benefit enormously from the advice, input and support of an educational supervisor. Every department should have a named and motivated person whose responsibility is managing the educational and developmental needs of any locum junior doctors based in their department.

The recent changes affecting International Medical Graduates' (IMG) access to training programmes in the UK have produced an isolated and worried cohort of trainees. Many have opted to take non-career grade posts from August 2007 when faced with uncertainty about the number of training posts, permit-free training and the changing status of the highly skilled migrant programme visa.

Educational supervisors cannot anticipate government policy on IMGs but the trust's human resources department or the deanery can help with employment queries. It is likely that large numbers of recently appointed and relatively junior non-career grade doctors will seek out educational supervisors for their personal development and support in the coming years.

Assessments

Educational supervisors should be able to explain the ongoing assessment process for their specialty and the format the annual review takes. The educational supervisors must ensure that their trainees can produce the evidence for learning outcomes and competencies for that year of training. The trainees should make sure that all their paperwork is correct, and they should check in advance with their supervisor that there are no outstanding problems to be addressed and documented. The formal annual review

(Record of In-Training Assessment/RITA or Annual Review of Competence Progression/ARCP) is about reviewing a trainee's progress and ensuring that he or she has achieved that year's training goals. It is *not* about presenting the trainee with new concerns or evidence of failure that have not been explored with the trainee beforehand.

Dealing with the challenging trainee

If the educational supervisor is made aware of an area of concern by a colleague then a meeting with the trainee should be arranged as soon as is possible. This may lead to a resolution of any potential conflict before events escalate. The same rule of an early meeting applies when the trainee's performance has been outstanding in a particular situation. Feedback should be given as soon as possible after the event in order to be effective (Box 1.2).

Box 1.2

A trainee felt that his concerns about his salary were not being dealt with quickly enough by the deanery. He took to phoning the personnel officer concerned on a regular basis and then started sending daily e-mails. Despite being asked to stop, he continued this behaviour, which was on the point of being logged as harassment by the deanery when the trainee's educational supervisor became involved. A discussion and explanation between the trainee and his educational supervisor on ways to resolve the conflict followed and became a useful management learning exercise for the trainee. The threat of a complaint about the trainee was diffused by a more constructive and conciliatory approach and a more realistic time frame agreed for reviewing his salary.

The challenging trainee is the trainee who takes up a disproportionate amount of the educational supervisor's time. This includes trainees with attitude problems, communication difficulties, unrealistic expectations or bullying tendencies, and extends to trainees with serious psychiatric disorders.

An extremely important role for the educational supervisor is to be part of the mechanism for identifying problems early and being able to put in place the support mechanisms to prevent any further deterioration. Challenging trainees frequently lack insight into their own problems in terms of professional behaviour and performance and are unlikely to spontaneously seek help. If the educational supervisor is made aware of any performance outside the acceptable limits of practice, they must arrange a prompt meeting with the trainee.

Challenging trainees can be identified in many ways, often obvious in retrospect. Some of the most common signs are a change in attitude at work, deteriorating clinical performance, isolation from his or her peer group, increasing time off sick or turning up late for work. In the first instance the educational supervisor should set about information gathering, looking for signs and symptoms, along with any possible causes.

It is vital to remember – 'if it's not written down, it did not happen'. Serious concerns about a trainee from any quarter must be in writing and an ongoing log of accurate documentation when addressing the problem is essential. Any written statements should be shown to the trainee. The trainee's recollection of what was proposed or agreed at the conclusion of a meeting may be completely different from that of the educational supervisor. Ensure that the trainee reads through the contemporaneous notes and signs them to show agreement on any action plan. If the trainee disagrees with any of the aspects of your synopsis, he or she should be allowed to add comments, again signed and dated.

If a conflict is expected then a colleague should be asked to join the meeting during which feedback is given. A second colleague can also be extremely useful if reservations about a trainee relate to only to one area of practice. For example, if the area of concern relates to work on the intensive care unit (ICU) then having a consultant colleague from that area to explain the feedback and put it into context can assist in resolving these issues (Box 1.3).

Box 1.3

Nurses on the intensive care unit (ICU) voiced their concerns about a junior doctor taking decisions without seeking senior advice. An initial meeting with the educational supervisor failed to resolve the matter as the trainee refused to acknowledge that there was a problem. A second meeting with an ICU consultant present produced a more focussed discussion around documented incidents. It became apparent that the trainee did not understand the importance of involving the whole team in patient care decisions and that this included the nursing staff as well as senior colleagues.

A useful starting point, which indicates whether a problem is going to be easily addressed or not, is to ask the trainee to reflect on what he or she thinks is going well and whether he or she is aware of any issues or areas where improvement is needed. Lack of insight is not a simple problem to resolve. However, if not tackled early it can cause isolation from the peer group, fragment the function of the team and ultimately limit the individual's career progression.

Managing the challenging trainee requires time and commitment from both parties. The supervisor should endeavour to:
- Be supportive and non-judgmental;
- Try and maintain a positive outlook;
- Encourage a commitment to change;
- Try and identify common themes, for example communication skills and time management;
- Listen to the trainee;
- Consider 360° feedback if the trainee is not convinced that there is a problem;
- Direct the trainee towards suitable learning resources;
- Encourage reflection and
- Act as a role model by discussing his or her approach to a tricky situation.

After the discussion, there needs to be a specific agreed plan, with a target for assessment of progress. The trainee should be assured of confidentiality. *The educational supervisor must remember at all times that any breach of information gathered under the auspices of a confidential meeting is catastrophic for both parties.* Information should not be disclosed without prior permission of the trainee.

Personal experience suggests that at any time 1% of trainees may be in a disturbed state of mind, which may affect their ability to work, and another 5% will need additional support to prevent minor problems from escalating. This may be a recurrence of a previous problem, for example an acute exacerbation of a chronic depressive disorder, or a new, sudden loss of confidence in the workplace precipitated by an apparently minor event. A good prognostic sign is the trainee who seeks support early and is honest about his or her mental health.

The educational supervisor must be aware that any serious matter such as working under the influence of alcohol or drugs or undertaking work outside the trainee's sphere of competence, or any issue of patient safety, needs to be referred to higher authorities, for example the trust's human resources department and the deanery. This should be clearly explained to trainees so that they become part of any referral process. If trainees demonstrate their involvement in seeking assistance, those investigating an incident will view this as a positive response. The whole referral process can be a very difficult and emotionally draining experience for all involved.

A trainee who refuses to comply with recommended local resolution procedures following a serious incident or problem or after committing a criminal offence must be referred directly to the GMC [7].

Educational supervisors should not try to manage challenging trainees on their own. It is important that educational supervisors know where to seek advice and to whom a trainee should be referred. *Educational supervisors must be careful with trainees who have a psychiatric component to their problems.* The role of the educational supervisor is to facilitate the trainee in accessing appropriate support services, not to be the support service. It is very easy for an inexperienced and well-meaning educational supervisor to be completely overwhelmed and manipulated by a trainee.

Do educational supervisors make a difference?

The importance of supervision in its broadest sense is referred to in successive reports of the Confidential Enquiry into Peri-Operative Death, which indicate that clinical supervision is associated with a positive effect on patient outcome whereas lack of supervision is harmful to patients [8]. The purpose of supervision is to improve patient care. In their review of supervision in clinical practice, Kilminster and Jolly conclude that the quality of the supervisory relationship is probably the single most important factor for effective supervision rather than the method of supervision used [9]. There is published work from the United States looking at the benefits of direct supervision of residents in terms of quality of care in five Harvard teaching hospitals [10], but there remains very little theoretical basis for current supervisory practice and hardly any research into the quality of medical educational supervision.

A postal questionnaire of 129 paediatric specialty registrars in the North Thames Deanery in 2005 found the most useful aspects of the educational supervisory role to be:
• Feedback on performance;
• Career advice and
• Objective setting.
However, aspects universally commented upon as poor included:
• Commitment;
• Lack of protected time to meet;
• The need to listen rather than talk and
• The need to encourage.
In this survey a number of consultants remained unaware of what was required from them as an educational supervisor and the trainees' conclusions were that only committed consultants should become educational supervisors, otherwise it becomes a process which is not valued by the trainees [11]. Some of these concerns are mirrored by the findings of a review from five postgraduate centres in the UK pertaining to preregistration house officers at the beginning and end of their preregistration year where lack of protected time and perceived inconsistent support from educational supervisors was highlighted [12]. In contrast, trainees from across the Mersey Deanery in their second-year foundation programme reported positively on their interactions with educational supervisors, the benefits of which included career advice, setting objectives and assessing educational needs [6].

Why become an educational supervisor?

Every doctor in training should have an educational supervisor but not everyone is suitable to become one. Educational supervisors have to be interested in and want to be involved with supporting trainees. This can be a demanding, time-consuming and occasionally stressful responsibility.

The rewards are not immediate. However, watching a trainee succeed can be a positive experience for both the trainee and the supervisor and, in the longer term, a successful educational supervisor network raises the profile of a department and assists recruitment at all levels.

The postgraduate deans suggest that the role of educational supervisor should take the equivalent of 1 hour per trainee per week, this time being included within the existing consultant job plan under the umbrella of SPA. This may be insufficient in the face of more detailed trainee assessments being required of educational supervisors as part of competency-based training. There is no direct financial remuneration although the role of educational supervisor should be highlighted on a clinical excellence award form.

If being an educational supervisor inspires you, there are other educational roles to explore including college tutor, foundation or specialty programme director, regional adviser and other positions within your trust, college or specialist society (see further resources).

References

1. General Medical Council. The New Doctor 2007: standards for training which Foundation Programme course providers need to meet. GMC, London, 2007.
2. Butterworth T, Faugier J. Clinical supervision and mentorship in nursing. Chapman and Hall, London, 1992.
3. Owen JP. A survey of the provision of educational supervision in occupational medicine in the Armed Forces. Occup Med 2005; **55**: 227–233.
4. Royal College of Anaesthetists. CCT in anaesthesia I: general principles. A manual for trainees and trainers. RCA, London, 2007.
5. Brown J, Chapman T, Graham D. Becoming a new doctor: a learning or survival exercise? Med Educ 2007; **41 (July)**: 653–660.
6. O'Brien M, Brown J, Ryland I, Shaw N, Chapman T, Gillies R, Graham D. Exploring the views of second year Foundation Programme doctors and their educational supervisors during a deanery-wide pilot Foundation Programme. Postgrad Med J 2006; **82**: 813–816.
7. General Medical Council. Referring a doctor to the GMC: a guide for health professionals. GMC, London, 2006.
8. Caalum KG, Gray AJG, Hoile RW, Ingram GS, Martin IC, Sherry KM, Whimster F. Then and now – the 2000 Report of the National Confidential Enquiry into Perioperative Deaths. NCEPOD, London, 2000.
9. Kilminster SM, Jolly BC. Effective supervision in clinical practice settings. Med Educ 2000; **34**: 827–840.
10. Sox CM, Burstin HR, Orav EJ, Conn A, Setnik G, Rucker DW, Dasse P, Brennan TA. The effect of supervision of residents on quality of care in five university – affiliated emergency departments. Acad Med 1998; **73 (7)**: 776–782.
11. Lloyd B, Becker D. Paediatric specialist registrars' views on educational supervision and how it can be improved. Arch Child Disord 2005; **G217**: A77.
12. Doran T, Maudsley G, Zakhour H. Time to think? Questionnaire survey of pre-registration house officers' experience of critical appraisal in the Mersey Deanery. Med Educ 2007: **41 (5)**: 487–494.

CHAPTER 2

Personal support and mentoring

Judy McKimm
Centre for Medical and Healthcare Sciences, University of Auckland, Auckland, New Zealand

The role of the educational supervisor comprises a set of defined activities focussed on providing support to trainees which enables them to achieve their educational objectives. However, as with many teaching and learning roles, the supervisor's role often extends beyond simply ensuring trainees pass assessments and make appropriate career choices. Many young health professionals struggle: they can feel unsupported, isolated and under stress, not only because of the job but also because they are managing busy lives outside work. This is particularly relevant at times of transition and change, such as when starting the foundation programme, moving from one level to another, or when changing organisations or rotations. Providing timely and appropriate guidance and support can improve trainee retention and make training more fulfilling and enjoyable; it also facilitates professional development on the trainee's journey to independent medical practice.

This chapter considers aspects of supervision that concern trainees' and supervisors' needs in relation to the provision of personal support. We will look at the support educational supervisors may provide, such as guidance, counselling, advising, mentoring and coaching, and we consider some of the similarities and differences between these roles and activities. We define the boundaries and limitations of the support educational supervisors provide to trainees, when supervisors may need to seek help (for themselves or their trainees) and practical strategies for coping with and avoiding potentially difficult situations.

Some definitions

In this chapter, the term 'guidance' is used to mean a cluster of activities relating to facilitating decision-making about learning, clinical work or careers. The term 'support' refers to the wider aspects of learner or professional

Essential Guide to Educational Supervision in Postgraduate Medical Education.
Edited by Nicola Cooper and Kirsty Forrest. © 2009 Blackwell Publishing,
ISBN: 978-1-4051-7071-0.

support, which may include study skills, information technology skills, library services or academic support (for example evidence-based practice or advising on textbooks, protocols or articles relevant to learning more about clinical problems).

Here we focus on providing *personal support* to individual trainees in the course of educational supervision. Support and guidance often involve advising and acting as an advocate or mentor. Personal support may also entail using counselling skills, but not under the guise of offering a professional counselling service.

Personal support

This section will consider two aspects of personal support: the support that you as an educational supervisor provide to your trainees and the personal support that you may require for yourself.

What is personal support?

Depending on when you undertook your undergraduate medical course and subsequent professional experience, your experience of personal support in an academic or learning context may be very different from that which emerging medical graduates have experienced. This will influence trainees' expectations of your role as an educational supervisor; trainees may expect that someone will be formally available to discuss or dispense advice about personal aspects of their education and training.

Most undergraduate medical students will have been assigned a personal tutor, particularly in the early years of their programme. The role of the personal tutor is to provide an additional form of support for students as they start their new lives at university and begin to meet and work with patients, families, doctors and other health professionals. Personal tutors can provide an invaluable sounding board for students, offer advice on aspects such as study skills, and provide information on a range of services in and outside the medical school and university. The personal tutor role (sometimes called a pastoral role) also incorporates developing a personal relationship and rapport with the student so that a range of personal issues can be discussed (particularly those that may affect academic progress or professional development) within an organisational and professional context.

Principles underpinning personal support

In addition to educational guidance, supervisors are required to provide personal or pastoral support for trainee doctors. In the foundation programme, it falls within the organisation's area of responsibility to make sure that 'systems are in place to ensure appropriate support for the academic and welfare needs of foundation doctors' [1]. The primary purpose of providing personal support is to ensure the trainee achieves defined and agreed educational objectives; however, an approach to professional development that focuses on the whole person also includes a moral and legal duty of care towards the trainee.

Later in the chapter, we consider the boundaries related to personal support. Setting ground rules about your relationship is useful right from your first meeting with a trainee. This can form part of the 'learning contract' between you and the trainee. This contract might include frequency of meetings, how to make contact outside this arrangement, the structure of meetings, action planning and goal setting, an agreement around confidentiality and sharing of information, and a discussion about the rights, responsibilities and expectations of both you and the trainee. Although this may sound mechanistic and overly prescriptive, it can help you develop a relationship with your trainee that is grounded in mutual understanding and respect for one another's roles and needs.

One of the central principles underpinning the provision of effective personal support is empathy and the development of a good relationship with the trainee. It is useful to distinguish between empathy ('I feel your sadness') and sympathy ('I'm sorry for your sadness, I wish to help'). Here, basic counselling skills such as building rapport, breaking the ice, drawing the trainee out, listening, managing silence, clarifying, reflecting back, questioning, summarising, setting the target and managing closure are very useful. These skills must be grounded in a non-judgemental approach that allows enough challenge to ensure that trainees move along their journey and push their 'learning edges', but in a supporting and 'holding' way that encourages them to develop advanced competencies and ultimately take responsibility for their own learning and development. This approach needs to be coupled with academic and professional guidance and advice offering appropriate and timely information to the trainee. The supervisor must also be able to monitor progress, correct errors and suggest ways forward against formal assessments and the trainee's learning goals.

A number of techniques drawn from psychology, counselling and psychotherapy can be helpful in managing the supervisor–supervisee relationship. One of these is transactional analysis (TA), founded by Eric Berne [2], which includes many models relating to human interactions and communications. One model that can be helpful is that of the 'ego states'. Berne suggests that at any one time people function in one of three states: Parent (P), Adult (A) or Child (C), displaying characteristic behaviours that are grounded in feelings and emotions. Feelings and emotions that are based in past experiences are described as coming either from Parent (these parental messages are often phrases such as 'you must', 'you ought' or 'you should') or from the Child ego state (these may be inappropriate negative emotions such as fear, shame or worthlessness). In the supervision relationship, it is possible that Parent or Child ego states are invoked; however, the ideal ego state for both participants is that of Adult. Adult involves being 'in the moment' or the 'here and now', drawing on all one's available adult emotional resources and reasoning powers. Recognising when you or your supervisee may be in these ego states can provide a framework to explore and explain specific and repetitive areas of difficulty. It is essential that any exploration of this nature is undertaken in an Adult-to-Adult context.

Launer [3] suggests that 'certain themes arise again and again in the supervision literature, suggesting that there is a consensus around particular ideas that cross theoretical boundaries'. See Box 2.1.

Box 2.1

Supervisor and supervision themes identified by Launer [3, p. 18].

- Supervision should be about enabling, empowering and sustaining human values.
- Supervisors may need at different times to take on a variety of roles, including guide, advisor, role model, sponsor, teacher and facilitator.
- Supervision needs to pay attention to the personal, professional and relational aspects of the work.
- Supervisors always have to bear in mind three separate 'clients': the supervisee, the patient and the organisation.
- Supervision needs to address the complexity and uniqueness of the problems brought, in order to generate solutions or options that are the best fit.
- Supervision is an interactional process. To be effective, it depends on emotional attunement, mutual trust and usually an evolving relationship between the supervisor and the trainee.

Role boundaries

One of the key aspects of providing effective supervision is being able to manage role boundaries both within your role and also in relation to the roles and skills of others. Being realistic about what you can and cannot (and should and should not) do within the role is very important, recognising your professional and personal limits and boundaries. Reminding yourself that you cannot solve everything for the trainee and knowing when and to whom you should refer are helpful.

Although the distinctions between different roles and activities can often be very blurred in practice, being able to categorise and 'label' various aspects of your role in terms of educational supervision, clinical supervision, coaching, personal support or mentoring can be helpful for both you and your trainee.

Articulating what you think is happening in a meeting with a trainee can be a useful 'signposting' strategy. This can be done formally or with a little bit of humour – you will find your own style. You may like to think of yourself putting on different 'hats' as the conversation unfolds. De Bono's idea of the '6 thinking hats' suggests that people in a team can take on different ways of thinking (i.e. putting on different 'hats') to consciously adopt different positions on a topic [4]. This may be a helpful technique to use with trainees in that you might adopt various positions to engender different responses and promote different ways of thinking. You may say to the trainee, 'Let's look at the facts here ...' (white hat thinking); 'Let's look at some of the risks in your career suggestions' (black hat thinking); or 'You seem to be a bit negative on this point, let's look at the positive aspects and opportunities' (yellow hat thinking). Other ways of adopting different positions include taking on different roles, such as that of a counsellor, and using basic counselling skills and techniques (paraphrasing, clarifying, reflecting, active listening – 'It seems to me ...', 'It is almost as if ...') to encourage and facilitate a conversation.

Providing support through change and transition

As an educational supervisor, you will be working with trainees during periods of great change in their working patterns and professional relationships as they continue to develop their professional identities and competence. One of your key roles is to support trainees through these changes as they move towards independent practice.

Hay's model of the competence curve as a response to change (see Figure 2.1) reminds us that responses to change are similar to those during loss or bereavement [5]. Hay notes that as people move through the stages they will exhibit different behaviours and emotions. This can affect their competence, not only to perform tasks but also to engage with others. If trainees are undergoing personal change and stress (such as relationship breakdown, financial difficulties or moving house) as well as changing jobs or roles, then you may notice behaviours linked to personal stress or change, which can map onto the change curve.

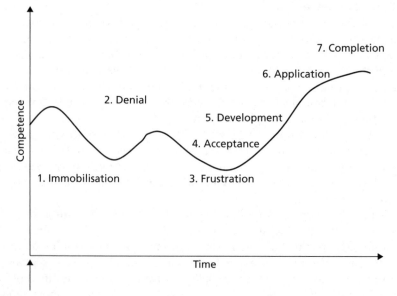

Figure 2.1 The response to change: the competence curve (Hay, 1996).

The list below describes the stages indicated in Figure 2.1 in more detail. As you read through this, try to identify how you as an educational supervisor could help a trainee move through these stages.

1. *Immobilisation – people seem to do nothing, to withdraw*
   This can be shown in behaviours such as absence due to minor illness, nonparticipation in additional activities over and above the daily workload or a lack of enthusiasm.

2. *Denial – a pretence that the change event has not happened*
   Here a trainee may stoically continue to perform at work whilst ignoring the emotional effects of a personal issue. People around the trainee notice a change in behaviour or personal appearance but the individual denies anything is wrong.

3. *Frustration – people know that they need to change but do not know how*
   An example of this stage may be where a trainee has had some negative feedback about his or her performance but has not been provided with enough information or support to make the required changes.

4. *Acceptance – people start exploring options that might be appropriate to the situation*
   Here your role might be to provide a forum and space for the trainee to discuss options with you or colleagues.

From here, your role has a different emphasis and the type of support you provide will be different. The next stages can be seen as plotting onto the novice to expert continuum as the trainee moves from 'unconscious incompetence to conscious incompetence to conscious competence to unconscious competence' [6].

5. *Development*
   New skills and knowledge are developed towards becoming a competent performer.

6. *Application*
   New skills are applied within the new identity.

7. *Completion*
   Here people have come through the transition and are no longer consciously aware of the change.

In a similar way in which patients and carers may respond to loss and bereavement, you may find your trainees looping back through the stages – it is not always a linear progression. In Figure 2.1, you can see that when people respond to change with immobilisation and frustration, they are at their lowest competence level. It may be a useful technique to use this model to raise awareness in the trainees of what may be happening. It can be particularly helpful to say to trainees that this is a normal response to change. If you know that your trainees are going through a major change, then it is also useful to note that their competence may be compromised at some point and to keep a more watchful eye on their progress or provide extra support.

Structuring meetings

Related to the relationship and interactional aspects of Launer's suggestions [3], you might structure every meeting with the trainee to end with an open question and subsequent discussion. For example you might say:

'OK, we have ten minutes left. Are there any aspects of the job that concern you or that you'd like help with? I'm thinking here particularly of how you're managing with [insert situation regarding context]'. For example:

• your mother being in hospital;
• just having changed jobs;
• moving house;
• starting your surgical rotation;
• (or whatever is appropriate to the individual trainee).

Allowing trainees the time and space to consider personal issues gives them permission to raise these issues with you. This technique acknowledges that the trainee has a life in which work and training are one (albeit important) element; it also allows you to connect with trainees on a deeper level and to develop an 'evolving relationship'. After you get to know the trainees, you may not need a specific time for discussing their personal issues. However, allocating the time sends trainees a good message – that you are there for them and are interested in them as a person rather than simply concerned about their role. It also helps you to carry out the dual activities of affirming your trainees (not only in terms of their decisions, relationships with others and assessment results, but also as a person) and challenging them about their performances, behaviours and impact on others.

Good supervision often pushes trainees out of their comfort zone so that they can learn, explore ideas and possibilities, and make changes to their practice. This calls for fine judgement. For some trainees, challenge can provoke anxiety, defensiveness and stress, particularly if personal issues or interpersonal dynamics are impeding professional performance and development. Being able to consciously switch from a formal style to a more relaxed and open style through your posture, positioning vis-à-vis the trainee, the words you use and the tone of your voice can help to challenge and extend the trainee and explore the aspects that may be uncomfortable and difficult. Setting aside time at the end of the session for discussion about the trainee's personal issues can provide a much needed space for repair and recovery.

Another way of structuring a meeting and developing a safe environment is to formally have on- and off-the-record conversations. Here, the formal aspects of the meeting may be recorded with action points and goals signed off by you and the trainee. The more personal aspects can be off record and not recorded on the trainee's file. The off-record conversations might be at the start or the end of a meeting. Issues that trainees may want to discuss with you in confidence and that may have no specific and immediate impact on their job performance or studies might include a relationship break-up, a long and drawn-out house move, care for elderly parents or financial worries.

Personal support and confidentiality

The Postgraduate Medical Education Training Board (PMETB) standards for training for the foundation programme [1] emphasise that the primary concern of those supporting junior doctors (including educational supervisors) is to ensure patient safety, stating that 'all those who teach, supervise, give counselling to, employ or work with foundation doctors are responsible for protecting patients. Patients will be protected through explicit and accountable supervision'. This, of course, applies to all postgraduate trainees. If this is clearly stated at the outset of the supervising relationship in the form of a contract, then all parties are protected.

Difficulties that trainees may present with include those related to health (infection, stress, substance misuse and mental illness), performance (unprofessional conduct both within and outside the workplace), workplace (long hours, bullying and harassment, and dysfunctional teams), and work–life balance or personal issues. These issues may be categorised as relating to 'doctors in difficulty' and are discussed in more detail in Chapter 3. A key point to note is that 'those responsible for training have a responsibility to share information with relevant individuals about [trainee] doctors that is relevant to their development as a doctor ... where possible the doctor should agree to this. Where the doctor does not agree, or is not able to do so, those responsible for training must consider the doctor's rights to confidentiality and any serious risk posed to patients, the public, themselves or colleagues when deciding to share information with other people involved in training the doctor' [1].

This raises questions about what constitutes personal information and what does not, and also highlights where boundaries concerning professional confidence lie.

A useful way of thinking about professional confidence in relation to your trainee is to think about it in the same way as you would regarding information that patients tell you. Some of this has direct relevance to their health or clinical condition, and is recorded in their notes and may be shared with health professionals. Other information they tell you is interesting and helps you understand them better but does not relate specifically to their condition or recovery. You probably would not record this in the notes. If you thought a trainee was a risk to him or herself or to others, or if you felt that other people needed to know something about the trainee for his or her own well-being, then you would tell other people about this so that something could be done, with the trainee's consent, agreement and knowledge in most cases, but not in extreme or crisis situations.

You will need to judge for yourself how much you want to encourage trainees to discuss their personal lives and what you think the impact may be on their work. Clearly trainees may raise personal issues with you that have a direct bearing and consequence on their medical practice and that cannot be off-record.

It is helpful to remember that you are not alone when dealing with a trainee who might pose a risk, and knowing who you should formally turn to for advice and guidance if such a situation arises is vital. Thankfully such situations are rare, but if they do arise you will need to make it absolutely clear to the trainee what you perceive is going on, what you plan to do about it, what the implications are for the trainee and his or her work, and what the specific next steps would be.

A situation may arise as a consequence of information having been passed onto you by others, in which case your role may be to convey bad news. It may be that a trainee discloses information that you feel is so serious in terms of potential risks that you need to share it in a formal way with others. It is very important in this case that you try to gain the trainee's consent to share the information, while making it clear that if he or she does not agree, your primary responsibility and duty of care as an educational supervisor is to ensure patient safety. When this conflicts with your responsibility to your trainee then patient safety is paramount. When someone discloses such a piece of information, one of the key signposting phrases is 'I need to stop you there …' and state what your position is in relation to what the trainee just told you. For example, 'Given what you have just told me, I need to explain that I have serious concerns that your behaviour (etc) poses a risk to patients and that I need to share this information with (whoever) …'. You can then go on to seek consent and explain the next steps. This will require you to know and be able to explain and provide information on the formal procedures within your organisation and possibly also with the Deanery or General Medical Council (GMC).

A summary of practical steps that you can take when working with a trainee in response to problematic behaviours or inappropriate attitudes is shown in Box 2.2 [7].

Box 2.2

Summary of practical steps that you can take when working with a trainee in response to problematic behaviours or inappropriate attitudes [7].
- Seek evidence of insight – in the light of professional expectations, on the effect and impact on patients, colleagues and carers and understanding the reasons they behaved in the way they did.
- Offer specific feedback – as soon as possible after the event, asking for their views and understanding, being specific about the examples cited and verbatim quotes of what was said, and working with the trainee to identify behaviours that can be changed. For example, 'The way in which you express your religious beliefs is offensive to some patients' is preferable to, 'The problem is your religious beliefs'.
- Refer to social, legal and professional norms – know what these are and provide evidence if needed, explain how the attitude or

(Continued)

> **Box 2.2** (Continued)
>
> behaviour conflicts with acceptable practice and identify in your own
> mind your particular prejudices and the influence of these on your
> actions.
>
> - Encourage and model reflective practice – this requires a degree of
>   openness that may be unfamiliar and threatening. Share examples of
>   encounters with patients that did not go as well as they should, thus
>   modelling reflective thinking and practice with the trainee.
> - Look for underlying problems – are there any extenuating circum-
>   stances for the attitude or behaviour that may require further help
>   such as counselling?
> - Document – keep a formal written record of discussions, correspond-
>   ence and your own recommendations; make sure you are aware of
>   who needs to know information and when; share the documentation
>   with the trainee, who may wish to disagree in writing, although this
>   does not mean that your documentation is invalid.
> - Seek further help – this is necessary in some circumstances and may
>   depend on the degree of inappropriateness of the behaviour or atti-
>   tude or its effect on patients or colleagues. Find out about sources of
>   help, for the trainee and for yourself.
> - Look for evidence of change – document this and share information
>   across disciplines and contexts as appropriate.

Self-care

The personal support aspects of being an educational supervisor can be
extremely varied and at times emotionally demanding. It is very important
that you identify your own support structures and use them when you need
to. Later in the chapter we look at two possible organisational support mechanisms: mentoring and action learning. However, one of the most important
ways in which you can remain effective is by developing and implementing
self-support and self-supervision techniques. This involves knowing yourself, developing self-insight and spotting when things that trainees say or
do press your own emotionally sensitive spots. These skills are very similar to those we use with patients: being mindful, listening to our inner conversations, recognising our somatic and emotional responses to situations
and developing a 'parallel dialogue' or 'reflection in action' (see Chapter 7)
through which we offer moment-to-moment supervision of our actions,
words and behaviours.

Earlier in the chapter, we looked at the range of roles and skills that might
be useful in offering personal support to trainees. These include communication skills, counselling skills, time management, managing structured meetings, educational or professional guidance, goal setting, coaching, providing

information, identifying options and knowing about referral agencies or individuals. It is likely that you will identify training needs as you take on such roles. This might be on-the-job development such as finding out more information about structures or people within the organisation or attending a training course to develop your counselling skills or advanced communication skills.

For your own protection, you need to walk the line between maintaining confidentiality and potentially colluding with a trainee to cover up something that impacts on his or her work. It is far safer to maintain a formal professional role and keep information recorded somewhere, even if it is a personal file note, or discuss options with an appropriate colleague, than to keep the matter entirely to yourself. This highlights another aspect of personal support in relation to the duty of care that you have not only for a trainee but also for yourself.

Another danger area when discussing personal issues with trainees is that you may cross another boundary and unwittingly become a trainee's main confidante and friend. This might happen if you are a good listener, have an open-door policy and are sympathetic (as opposed to empathic) and caring. These are all good qualities for an educational supervisor, but need to be tempered with a watchful eye on the boundaries and expectations from your own professional role, the time you have available and the appropriateness of the conversations. This is particularly important when people are in a vulnerable emotional state. Attachments can easily become disproportionately intense and even sexual in nature, and can turn into resentment or anger, as when a trainee feels that you have been unwilling to act or advocate on his or her behalf or disagrees with something you have done. This can cause problems for both the trainee and yourself and needs to be nipped in the bud so that you can put the relationship back on a professional footing or pass the case on to a colleague.

It can be difficult if the relationship between you and your trainee breaks down temporarily or permanently; it is easy to take this as a personal failure. Again, it is important that you have someone to discuss this with, to talk about what has happened and whether there are any learning points for you.

As an educational supervisor you will understand the training programme (including changes to structure and assessments), the organisation, how it functions and your trainees. You will also need to know:
- The key personnel in the organisation and how to contact them.
- Details of the programme content.
- How progression and performance are recorded and your role in this (e.g. log books, personal development plans).
- Details of the main assessments relating to trainees.
- Details of support services for referral – these may include occupational health, counselling, voluntary/charity organisations and study support (e.g. for a dyslexic trainee).

There are two inter-related aspects of supervision that can cause anxiety and worry for supervisors: knowing when and to whom to refer trainees with difficulties and knowing when and from whom to ask for help when you are struggling in your role.

This highlights the need for educational supervisors to know their own capabilities and limitations and the professional and institutional boundaries within which they are working. It raises the question of, 'Who supervises the supervisors?' There is a range of formal and informal networks that help to provide support for supervisors. This will vary depending on your professional context and specific organisational structures, but may include colleagues (seniors and peers), other health professionals, agencies, services, royal colleges, deaneries, the British Medical Association and the General Medical Council.

Mentoring

'Mentoring is usually understood as guidance and support offered by a more experienced colleague' [3]. In this sense, mentoring is not dissimilar to some of the aspects of personal support we discussed in the preceding text. However, mentoring typically has other distinguishing features. There are aspects of mentoring that can provide useful frameworks or approaches for providing personal support for trainees.

Mentoring is usually distinguished from coaching in that coaching normally focuses on a limited number of tasks or a more complex task such as management or leadership development. Coaching often enables individuals to achieve personal or life fulfilment particularly at times of change or decision-making. A mentor helps another person to become what that person aspires to be – or, as the Standing Committee on Postgraduate Medical and Dental Education (SCOPME) notes, it is someone who 'guides another individual (the mentee) in the development and re-examination of their own ideas, learning and personal and professional development' [8].

The Homeric concept of the mentor is that of a wise counsellor, trusted friend and role model. A mentor can also be seen as a guide or a critical friend. This concept has been used in many organisational contexts, both formally and informally, to enable individuals who are new to an organisation or role to be inducted. Mentoring is usually seen as a one-to-one relationship, although there are also examples of peer-mentoring, co-mentoring and group mentoring. In some organisations, formal mentoring schemes are in place for new staff or staff who are moving into more senior positions. On other occasions, it is only through hindsight that individuals realise that they have been mentored, that someone has had a strong influence on their lives and careers or that particularly strong support has been provided at a time of difficulty or transition.

The idea of mentoring can be very helpful in relation to your own role with a trainee or regarding your own needs, particularly if you are new to educational supervision or new to an organisation. Your trust or practice may have a mentoring scheme in place in which you can participate, or you may find it helpful to identify someone who can act as your mentor. Mentoring relationships work best when there has been some choice, because compatibility and understanding are key to the success of the relationship. As in any support relationship that develops over time, the mentor initially may have a more supportive and guidance role within a safe and protected environment. As time goes on and the mentee develops confidence and becomes less dependent and more autonomous, the mentor can take on a more challenging, analytical, reflective and critical role.

A good mentor brings experience, perspective, objectivity and some distance into the mentoring relationship. He or she also offers empathy, honesty and openness. One of the strengths of the experience is that mentors can offer a long-term view about the profession, the organisation and the individual. They are influential in helping the individuals reach their goals or aspirations and are willing to share their expertise and experience.

Hay views the mentoring relationship as a 'life cycle' with four stages [9]:
- Stage 1 – initiation, orientation or courtship – creating an alliance, bonding, setting objectives (contracting) and defining an agenda.
- Stage 2 – honeymoon, getting established, adolescence, dependency and nurturing.
- Stage 3 – maturing, developing autonomy or independence.
- Stage 4 – ending, termination, divorce – closure and mourning.

This concept can be used with your trainee as you plan the sequence of meetings throughout your time together, recognising that the 'journey' will go through these stages. It is particularly important to manage closure and endings well, especially if you have worked on personal issues with the trainee. Although the supervisor–supervisee relationship may include some features of mentoring, and your trainee will see you as a role model, this brings to light one of the other aspects of your relationship with the trainee: that of power.

Power

As an educational supervisor you are in a position of power over your trainee and it is essential that you do not misuse or abuse that power, as this can undermine the relationship. There are many differences that may exacerbate an imbalance of power such as gender, age, race/ethnicity or culture, class, sexuality, seniority, qualifications, disability, speech/accent, parenthood or domestic responsibilities. Being aware of these potential power imbalances is important so that the supervisor can think about and address the impact these might have on the trainee. For example, trainees may behave defensively or become over-compliant and accept any ideas the supervisor suggests. Conversely, you may find yourself feeling challenged or deskilled by certain trainees due to implicit power imbalances.

Action learning for peer learning and support

Definitions

One form of support that is being used increasingly in education and professional development is action learning. This is when a group of people agree to work together in a mutual support structure (the action learning set) to explore issues and find more creative solutions to management and organisational challenges. The set members learn from helping each other, gaining greater skills in listening, questioning, diagnosing, coaching, role playing and creative problem solving. 'Action learning is a method of problem solving for managers which also offers scope for personal learning and development. The manager prepares for taking action on the job and at the same time learns about her/himself as a manager and as a person' [10].

Action learning has some similarities with other peer and professional support methods such as learning circles, Balint groups (meetings typically used by general practitioners to discuss difficult or intriguing cases) or social work supervision groups. However, action learning sets have a specific purpose, structure and process that distinguishes them from other methods' structures. Action learning can be a useful form of support for groups of professionals who have similar roles or jobs, such as educational supervisors, and who wish to share experiences and receive insightful comments about issues or problems. See Box 2.3 for the principles and ground rules of action learning sets.

Box 2.3

Principles and ground rules for action learning sets:
- There has to be total confidentiality and trust among set members.
- Members must feel it is safe to admit need and take risks.
- Members need to be able to try out new ways of relating, knowing that they will get constructive feedback and not be blamed for getting it wrong.
- Members need to get over any notion of competitiveness or being 'better than'.
- Members need to all sign up to the idea of a learning community/ community of practice.
- Members need to challenge one another and themselves as critical friends.
- Members should say 'I' – rather than saying 'One', 'We' or 'You' when they mean 'I'. This helps to ensure that everyone owns his or her statements.
- Members should actively listen to one another and give each other space.
- The set members' role is enabling, not advising – members are to help the issue holder find his or her best course of action, not offer their own solutions, unless asked to as part of generating possibilities.

The purpose of action learning sets is to enable each person to develop capabilities, direction, challenge situations and their own personal style and to help set members 'solve' real-life problems and learn from doing so [11]. The core of action learning is the process of learning from and with others, rather than actually solving the problem. A typical set would have between five and eight members, enough to generate a dialogue and discussion but not so many that members do not get individual turns with their 'issue' or 'problem'.

An action learning set may have a negotiated process between set members, but usually a set will appoint a convenor to keep time and ensure people adhere to the ground rules. This role usually rotates around set members. It is important to keep to the external and internal time boundaries to ensure each person has a fair share of the time available. At the first meeting, ground rules are agreed. At each meeting a quick 'round' or 'check in' allows people time to say how they are, offer a recent highlight, report on what has happened since the last meeting and say what they want from the session. What people want out of the session forms the agenda.

Action learning sets structure

A typical structure of an action learning set would be:

- The members check in.
- The people who had the issues last time report back on what they did, noting what worked (no matter how small), what did not (where they got stuck) and what they need help with today (this may be a continuation of the old case or new case).
- The set agrees division of time and assigns a time keeper. Everyone needs to be an issue holder at some point; taking turns is important.
- The set takes each of the selected issues in turn (typically two or three in an hour and a half session) to help the owners see the case differently and/or their relationship to it, so that they get to the 'action step'.
- At the close of the session, everyone shares what 'I' have valued about the group today and/or an individual, and arrangements are made for the next meeting.

How does each person work through the issue with the rest of the set members?

Only one person at a time is the issue holder. For that time, the set members are there to listen and enable. If the problem owner is not getting the sort of help that is needed, he or she should say so. People are listened to without interruption as they recount their three-step story – this is another important ground rule. They first describe the situation or problems with which they want help. Then they express any feelings they have in relation to the situation. Finally they restate the problem; however, this time the problem owner includes a definition of what a positive outcome must include. Envisioning a creative, positive outcome is the first step towards realising it. Then the set members work with the issue holder to help him or her explore the resources available for tackling this problem [12].

Typical questions that set members might ask include:
• Who knows? Who has the necessary information?
• Who can help you? Who has the necessary skills?
• Who will help you? Who will give necessary support, political or otherwise?
• Who cares? Who will be affected by the changes involved?

It is important to avoid too much anecdotal comment or other set members' parallel problems ('I have a similar problem in my department ...'). This sounds quite a mechanistic process, but the structure and ground rules enable the process and sharing of issues to work well. As sets mature and start working well together, they may modify the process and work in different ways. Action learning is a proven method of helping participants learn while tackling real-life problems or issues, but set members must feel the need to make personal and professional changes. You can only learn about action learning and its value by actually engaging in it and actively participating.

Summary

Providing effective personal support for trainees is often challenging but should always be rewarding. It requires an open approach with your trainee within clearly agreed boundaries so that you both understand the expectations from the relationship. The supervisor–trainee relationship should enable mutual 'emotional and intellectual trust so that (trainees) can reflect frankly on their own work and learn continually' [3]. Working with your trainee in this holistic way echoes the partnership and empowerment approach that doctors are increasingly taking with their patients, and leads to more fulfilling educational supervision.

References

1. Postgraduate Medical Education and Training Board (PMETB)/General Medical Council. Standards for Training for the Foundation Programme, 2007. www.pmetb.org.uk/fileadmin/user/QA/QAFP/Standards_for_Training_270307.pdf [accessed 14 March 2008]
2. Berne E. Games people play: the psychology of human relationships. Grove/Atlantic Imported, 1964.
3. Launer J. Supervision, mentoring and coaching: one-to-one learning encounters in medical education. Association for the Study of Medical Education, Edinburgh, 2006.
4. De Bono E. Six thinking hats. The de Bono Group. http://www.debonogroup.com/6hats.htm [accessed 13 March 2008]
5. Hay J. Transactional analysis for trainers. Sherwood Publishing, Watford, UK, 1996.
6. Proctor B. Training for supervision: attitude, skills and intention. In: Cutliffe J, Butterworth T, Proctor B (Eds), Fundamental themes in clinical supervision. Routledge, London, 2001.
7. Martin J. Facilitating professional attitudes and professional development. Teaching and learning in clinical contexts: a resource for health professionals.

London Postgraduate Deanery website: www.clinicalteaching.nhs.uk 2003, [accessed 14 March 2008]

8. Standing Committee on Postgraduate Medical and Dental Education (SCOPME). Supporting doctors and dentists at work: an enquiry into mentoring. SCOPME, London, 1998.
9. Hay J. Transformational mentoring. McGraw-Hill, New York, 1995.
10. Gaunt R. Personal and group development for managers: an integrated approach through action learning. Longman, London, 1991.
11. Brockbank I, McGill A. The action learning handbook: powerful techniques for education, professional development and training. Routledge Falmer, Oxford, 2004.
12. Reavons R. The ABC of action learning. Chartwell-Bratt, Bromley, Kent, 2003.

CHAPTER 3

Doctors in difficulty

Rosalind Roden
Yorkshire and the Humber Postgraduate Deanery; ATLS® Steering Group,
The Royal College of Surgeons of England, London

Doctors in general are slow to recognise or accept that they are experiencing difficulties in their careers. Historically, doctors have felt they should work hard to maintain a professional reputation that demonstrates no weakness or shortcomings. The almost god-like reverence with which doctors were regarded until recent years did nothing to help doctors recognise when there were problems with their conduct or careers. It was almost regarded as a sign of 'poor moral fibre' for a doctor to admit that he or she was experiencing difficulties; even if a doctor realised there was a problem, there was often limited access to available resources that could help.

As a result, doctors who were failing to succeed for whatever reason were generally ostracised and frequently counselled into different careers. Only rarely was there an opportunity for doctors to feel supported in overcoming their difficulties. The dawn of a new generation of trainers interested in good medical education, including the welfare of doctors in training, has fortunately changed this. There are now excellent mechanisms in place for identifying doctors who are in difficulty. However, even now, some of these doctors will still fail to be recognised and there may be a delay in their receiving advice and guidance.

Helping a doctor in difficulty can be a challenging and demanding task. This chapter explains how we as educational supervisors can help our colleagues who are in difficulty. It starts with a description of the different reasons why doctors may be in difficulty and how to recognise them, and then describes in general and specific terms how to proceed. It also outlines the resources that are available for continuing help and support.

Essential Guide to Educational Supervision in Postgraduate Medical Education.
Edited by Nicola Cooper and Kirsty Forrest. © 2009 Blackwell Publishing,
ISBN: 978-1-4051-7071-0.

What is 'a doctor in difficulty'?

A significant minority of doctors find themselves in difficulty at some stage in their careers. Failure to tackle problems or inappropriate management of them may have long-term consequences for the doctor and may jeopardise patient safety. All of us involved in the training of doctors must be able to recognise colleagues in difficulty and help them seek prompt and effective management at an early stage.

Health problems

While doctors are trained to recognise and treat ill health in their patients, they can be poor at recognising problems with their own health. As a consequence, a doctor with health problems can be one of the most difficult situations to deal with. Frequently there is a denial of the health problem, failure to seek correct treatment and a lack of insight as to whether or not the individual is well enough to continue working.

Doctors are vulnerable to exactly the same health problems that affect the rest of the population. In addition, there are problems that may be related to the lifestyle and workplace risks that doctors are exposed to, including stress and infections. In general, physical health problems are easier to recognise and deal with.

Because of the undeniable stigma associated with mental health problems, illnesses such as depression and anxiety in doctors can be far more challenging to deal with than physical problems. The basis of helping doctors with mental health problems is to accept that these problems do exist and can be successfully treated, and ensure that they do not preclude doctors from continuing in their careers.

Performance problems

Most doctors would agree, if they thought carefully about it, that at some stage in their career they have had a 'performance problem'. For the majority, this would be a situation in which they felt their knowledge was not as good as it should have been, their clinical judgement was not as sharp as they would have wished or their practical skills were not as fine tuned as they would have hoped.

Perception of failing to perform as expertly as one would wish is a relatively common trait in the medical profession. However, performance becomes an issue when there is a *sustained* failure in performance, which begins to affect either patients' welfare or colleagues in the workplace. Significant performance problems centre around knowledge, skills or attitudes. In general, the first two of these are far easier to deal with than the third.

The new assessment and appraisal structures in postgraduate medical education mean that performance is now more formally monitored, and therefore underperforming doctors, in theory, are much easier to identify and support. The most important aspect of this is to ensure that problems are dealt with in a timely fashion and by a correct mechanism.

Conduct problems

Conduct problems can be divided into issues within the workplace and those outside the workplace. Both may be equally serious and have a significant effect on a doctor's career progression.

Conduct problems within the workplace most often take the form of rudeness, laziness or indiscretion with colleagues or patients. In the past, doctors displaying such traits were often regarded as being of a 'certain stereotype'. The famous 'Doctor in the House' films portrayed Sir Lancelot Spratt shouting and bullying his juniors, and this was regarded as almost normal behaviour. The realisation that this is not acceptable has been a giant step in managing conduct problems among doctors.

All of us have felt ourselves in a situation in which our anger is rising, and found it difficult to stop ourselves from saying something we know we would regret later. Most of us, however, would be able to control our emotions in a difficult situation. A small minority of doctors believe that it is acceptable to lose their temper with patients or colleagues.

Other forms of unprofessional conduct, such as laziness or poor time-keeping, can have a significant impact on colleagues. The golden rule is to work alongside one's colleagues as a team. It is difficult to welcome a team member who is constantly missing work or turning up late. Inevitably these doctors become unpopular and, in turn, this can make their conduct worse.

The greatest issue with conduct problems is lack of insight. Many doctors who are behaving in an unprofessional manner do not see this in themselves. Many feel that they are conscientious, hard-working individuals whose occasional outbursts of temper or rudeness are permissible given the responsibilities and challenges of their job.

Unprofessional conduct outside the workplace is also a serious issue. Because of the duties of a doctor, those acts that are considered dishonest, fraudulent or criminal will be brought to the attention of the General Medical Council (GMC). This is perhaps one of the most complex situations for an educational supervisor to deal with. Establishing accurate facts and maintaining confidentiality are important in the early stages of this process.

Workplace problems

Workplace problems are becoming more frequent and a greater contributing factor for doctors finding themselves in difficulties. Excessive hours or work intensity are becoming a thing of the past but many doctors, particularly in senior positions, still find themselves, either by choice or by necessity, working longer hours than would be considered reasonable by other professions. In addition, inadequate resources such as staffing, equipment or facilities may contribute to a doctor experiencing persistent difficulties at work, which begin to affect his or her performance.

One of the most serious and intimidating workplace problems is bullying. Bullying, to a greater or lesser extent, has been accepted in medical education in the past. Sometimes it is obvious to others around; other times it is more subtle and may only be apparent to those directly involved. Being bullied leads to lack of confidence, misery at work and, frequently, underperformance. Wherever a doctor has been found to be underperforming there should be a careful review to ensure that bullying is not part of the problem.

Bullying may take the form of intimidation, public criticism, humiliation or inconsistent expectations. Doctors may be expected to work outside their contract of employment, and if they object to this, they may find their position is threatened. The worst types of bullying may involve racism or sexism. These are often the hardest to identify, and in many cases, the subject of the bullying will deny it is occurring because they feel frightened or embarrassed. Very often those who are being bullied feel that things will get worse if the attention of others is drawn to it.

Work–life balance problems

Doctors are good at separating their home and work lives and preventing 'minor' domestic problems from affecting their performance at work. However, it is not always possible to do this consistently, particularly when personal problems become a major issue.

Certain situations, such as the illness of a close family member or friend, may have a significant effect on a doctor's performance. There may be practical issues such as the need to attend outpatient clinics or to care for an unwell relative. There may also be emotional problems, in particular feelings of guilt and helplessness, that the doctor is abandoning a family member to go to work. Finally, there may be issues at work that become unexpectedly upsetting for a doctor because they are reminiscent of a situation that is occurring at home. Other personal problems such as financial difficulties, divorce or geographical separation from a loved one may also affect a doctor's performance.

Although this chapter lists the different types of difficulties doctors may encounter, very often doctors in difficulty experience a combination of the above-mentioned problems. Many difficulties are interrelated. For example, a doctor who has domestic problems may find it difficult to study for examinations or work long shifts or at weekends. He or she may often be late for work, and find themselves short tempered or abrupt with colleagues or even patients. Failure in examinations may lead to even lower levels of confidence and performance, and in turn to frustration from a supervisor. If there is a failure to identify the *initial* problem, the way the failing doctor is dealt with may go on to magnify the issues rather than deal with them.

Managing a doctor in difficulty

General principles

Doctors in difficulty come to the attention of their seniors or educational supervisors in a number of ways. Sometimes doctors themselves will ask for help; sometimes attention is drawn to the problem by failure to complete examinations or projects. Occasionally there is a trend of worrying concerns noticed by other professionals who work with the doctor. Complaints, either written or verbal, from patients or relatives may also be a catalyst that alerts an educational supervisor to the fact that a doctor is experiencing difficulties.

Depending on the problem, the process will vary. However, there are certain principles of good practice that underpin the process of managing any doctor in difficulty.

All discussions with the doctor concerned should take place in an appropriate and *confidential* environment. A doctor's difficulties should never be discussed with colleagues without the doctor's permission, and never in the clinical setting or in front of patients or relatives. Discussions with others may be necessary as part of a formal process to help the doctor.

Honesty and confidentiality are vital at all times. It is likely that there will be differing opinions from the doctor and from those who have generated the concerns. Whoever is in the position of managing the process must be aware that he or she should remain impartial at all times – this is particularly important during the early stages when information is being gathered. On many occasions, things are not what they seem initially. One of the common mistakes made by supervisors is to act on the statements of one individual. See Box 3.1 for the 'Ten Commandments' for dealing with doctors in difficulty.

Box 3.1 The 'Ten Commandments' for managing doctors in difficulty

- Listen
- Be honest
- Be realistic
- Do not judge
- Document discussions
- Set goals and time limits
- Maintain confidentiality
- Involve those who really need to know
- Use other resources
- Offer support – doctors in difficulty are lonely

The cornerstone of managing a doctor in difficulty is *documentation and communication*. In the past, poor documentation, or in many cases a complete lack of documentation, has been the main contributor to failure to manage a doctor in difficulty. It is important to communicate, while maintaining confidentiality, with those who need to be involved in the process of helping the doctor, such as the training programme director or postgraduate dean.

All documentation should be clearly and accurately recorded. Often it is helpful to document what was actually said by individuals, particularly if colleagues or patients have made statements about a doctor's performance or conduct. Statements can then be discussed with the doctor and his or her responses recorded.

Documentation should be as structured as possible and contain:
- a list of the concerns raised regarding the doctor's behaviour or conduct;
- details of situations and dates on which these concerns were raised;
- the doctor's own perception of the situation and what he or she regards as the problems;
- ways to manage the difficulty and the actions needed to be taken by both the doctor and the educational supervisor;
- any processes such as a period of targeted training, or other sources that the doctor has been asked to contact, for example occupational health or counselling sessions;
- any targets or outcomes that seem appropriate to document at that stage;
- a summary of what has been discussed including the actions that are to be taken by the trainee and/or the educational supervisor.

Whether the problem is to do with health, performance or conduct, if it is felt that there is a serious risk to patients or there has been a serious breach of trust, then the doctor should be suspended pending further investigation. This is a difficult action to take, and if it is necessary, ensure that the doctor is aware this is for safety reasons and is not a prejudgement of the outcome of an investigation.

Only the medical director or his appointed deputy can suspend a doctor, unless it is an absolute emergency. The National Clinical Assessment Service (NCAS) should be consulted prior to the suspension of any doctor. If the doctor is in training, the postgraduate dean must be informed.

When doctors have been suspended pending an investigation, support must always be offered. If the doctor is to be allowed to return to work then his or her duties may need to be modified. If a doctor has been suspended for several weeks, he or she will require a graded return to work under supervision until knowledge and skills have been re-established and confirmed.

Managing health problems

The approach taken will depend on the severity of the issue, but kindness and compassion are fundamental. Nobody wants to be ill. For physical conditions, for example an injury that requires time off work, the process can be relatively simple. It is essential that the doctor ensures certification (to the human resources department or the employer), and this requires regular contact with the doctor's general practitioner. If the condition is likely to have ongoing or permanent effects then it may be necessary to involve occupational health at an early stage. A referral can be made by the Trust or via the deanery if the doctor is in training. Once a doctor has been assessed by the occupational health department it may be necessary to involve human resources and/or the postgraduate dean. It may be that the doctor requires a graded return to work, alterations in the environment of the workplace or some more permanent adjustment such as less than full-time work or training. See Box 3.2 for the criteria for less than full-time work or training.

Box 3.2 Less than full-time training

Criteria for eligibility include:
- personal ill health (occupational health assessment);
- need to act as carer for unwell relative;
- child care (some deaneries will set an age limit for child/children);
- vocational need, for example to train in the church.

Other situations may be considered at the discretion of the local deanery. Job shares may be available for those not satisfying the eligibility criteria for supernumerary less than full-time training posts.

In a small number of cases, the injury or condition may preclude the doctor from returning to work in his or her previous capacity. A permanent physical disability does not mean that a doctor cannot return to work in a *different* capacity. Most deaneries have a number of people available to give advice regarding a change in medical careers or careers in general. Talking to those who can access resources and information can be enormously reassuring for a doctor who is facing the prospect of potential unemployment because of ill health.

Some health problems seem less serious in themselves but may dramatically affect performance. For instance, mental health problems such as mild depression, anxiety or stress may have a significant effect on a doctor's performance while not actually precluding them from the workplace. In general, a doctor's health problems should be initially dealt with by the general practitioner with appropriate referral to local specialists if necessary. When a period of sick leave becomes prolonged, it is important that some contact is maintained between the doctor and his or her educational supervisor, with involvement of occupational health if appropriate.

Occasionally doctors will not accept that they have a health problem. They may deny that their health issues are affecting their performance and may want to continue at work. If an educational supervisor feels that it is not in either the doctor's best interests or that of patients, steps must be taken to seek further help in order to advise the trainee. In this difficult situation the educational supervisor must inform the doctor of any concerns and explain that human resources and occupational health will need to be informed for an assessment. If the doctor is in postgraduate training then the postgraduate dean should also be informed. In the unusual situation of a doctor insisting on continuing to work despite significant health and performance problems it may be necessary to involve the GMC.

Substance misuse is a rare but extremely serious problem that may occasionally arise. If the substance misuse (e.g. alcohol excess or drug taking) is outside the workplace then it may be extremely difficult to establish the facts and persuade the doctor to seek advice. If a supervisor has significant concerns and feels that the doctor's performance at work is being affected then further advice must be sought from the trust or deanery.

Substance misuse occurring within the workplace, particularly if it involves drugs taken from the workplace, requires investigation by the employer and the police. Inevitably the doctor is suspended from work until a conclusion is reached. Significant substance misuse, particularly if it results in a criminal investigation, must be reported to the GMC and the postgraduate dean if the doctor is in training.

Managing performance problems

Performance problems in doctors can broadly be divided into problems with knowledge, skills or attitudes. A supervisor is sometimes alerted to a trainee or colleague's performance problems by the casual comments of others. It is important to differentiate comments that are based on facts and are well founded from those that may be because of personality clashes or different perceptions.

Obvious behaviours that might alert the trainer to difficulties include clinical mistakes; poor judgement; poor record-keeping; communication problems with patients, relatives or colleagues; failing professional examinations; or repeated or prolonged periods of absence because of sickness. Behaviours that may be less obvious include poor time-keeping or organisation, a change in appearance or emotional liability such as tearfulness or anger. Doctors who are hard to contact or fail to make arrangements for appropriate supervision or appraisals should also alert suspicion.

Performance problems that are identified and managed early are more likely to reach a satisfactory conclusion. It is also much easier to tackle a performance problem that the trainee agrees with and is aware of. Lack of insight magnifies the problem but can be resolved if handled correctly. See Box 3.3 for tips in managing those with lack of insight.

The first step is to establish whether there is a problem and what the problem is. This must always involve a direct discussion with the doctor concerned. There should also be detailed discussions with others directly

---

Box 3.3 Managing poor performance – dealing with lack of insight

- Explore in detail the doctor's progress over the last 12 months.
- Provide real examples/cases that demonstrate performance below standards.
- Provide statements from others.
- Talk through some clinical scenarios with the doctor: 'What would you do if...'.
- Suggest you observe the doctor in a clinical setting and give feedback.

involved, whether colleagues, patients or relatives. Accurate documentation is essential. Box 3.4 lists some statements that may help to introduce a problem.

Box 3.4 Managing poor performance – introducing the problem

- 'How do you think you are performing at the moment?'
- 'Do you feel you are making the right amount of progress?'
- 'Do you feel comfortable with your responsibilities?'
- 'Do you have any concerns about your work?'
- 'What do you think others think of your work?'

The supervisor must then make an assessment as to whether or not the performance problem carries a small risk or a significant risk to patients. It is also important to consider whether or not the performance problem is a result of a health or workplace issue (such as inadequate staffing or excessive hours of duty). If a performance problem is perceived as being of small risk then the next step is to formulate a written document between the supervisor and the doctor concerned (see Box 3.5).

Box 3.5 Managing poor performance – making a plan

- Document performance and standards that have not been achieved.
- Document evidence that these have not been achieved.
- Document action to address needs, and who is responsible for what.
- Document the assessment method of progress towards a target.
- Set a date for the review process.

A plan should include clear and concise documentation of what the problem is. It should also include evidence as to why the doctor is failing to achieve the required standard. The document should clearly record what steps the doctor needs to take to remedy the problem and how and when progress will be assessed. Both the doctor and the supervisor should retain copies of this document and both should sign it and agree to it.

While it is vital to respect confidentiality when dealing with performance problems, it is important even with those regarded as a small risk to inform the training programme director if the doctor is a trainee. If the doctor is expected to rotate to a different post it is also essential to inform the next educational supervisor.

More significant performance problems generally require a case conference. This should include the educational supervisor, a representative from human resources, the trainee and his or her supporter. It may also include the postgraduate dean or a representative. If the doctor is on a training programme then the training programme director should also be involved. A case conference should establish the facts and clearly establish what steps are needed to remedy the problem. A course of action must be agreed by both the doctor concerned and those at the case conference. Targets should be set with review dates.

Managing conduct problems

The procedure for managing a conduct problem is very similar to that for managing a performance problem; however if the conduct problem is significant, then outside agencies, including investigations by the police, may be necessary. If a more serious type of conduct problem such as dishonesty, fraud or theft is revealed then the medical director should be informed. If the doctor is in training, the postgraduate dean should be informed.

For conduct problems posing less of a serious risk, for example rudeness or laziness, there should be a clear discussion with the doctor. Health issues and workplace issues, especially stress, should also be considered. The nature of the conduct issue should be clearly documented. The steps taken to remedy the problem should also be documented with examples where possible. In particular it may be possible to arrange help such as mentoring or communication skills practice. There should then be a period of observation followed by a formal review. A date for this should be agreed.

Disciplinary procedures are the responsibility of the employing organisation, that is the healthcare trust, although in the case of a trainee there may be an agreement between the trust and the deanery as to who deals with such problems. The national framework for managing disciplinary problems in trainee doctors is laid out in the Department of Health document 'Maintaining High Professional Standards in the Modern NHS'.

Managing workplace problems

One of the most significant workplace problems encountered is bullying. This can be extremely difficult to manage because often the victim is reluctant to reveal the nature of the problem or seek help. Once a supervisor is aware that a colleague is being bullied, action must be taken. This must involve documented discussions with the doctor concerned first. A written statement of what has occurred is essential. Steps must be then taken to interview the person against whom the allegations have been made. It is particularly helpful in this circumstance to have the allegations in the form of written statements as they can then be discussed in detail.

If the allegations are substantiated then the medical director should be informed, and if the doctor is in training, the postgraduate dean must be informed. It is vital to ensure the safety of the doctor concerned and also ensure he or she has support. It may be necessary to review a doctor's place-ment particularly if it is felt that the doctor's performance may be affected by bullying. Bullying is an extremely serious offence and the employer may wish to take disciplinary action if bullying is proved. When possible, further action should include attempts to change the instigator's behaviour rather than extreme action, such as a dismissal or suspension.

Managing work–life balance problems

Managing work–life balance problems can be one of the most difficult areas to deal with. It is often difficult to establish that a doctor is having prob-lems outside the workplace that are affecting performance. Many doctors will attempt to hide such difficulties and feel that an admission of the prob-lem is an admission of failure. However, with the current system of regular appraisal for all doctors, work–life balance issues that may affect perform-ance are becoming easier to identify. Figure 3.1 can be used as part of a dis-cussion. While a doctor is entitled to keep his or her home life private and separate from work, if the issues are beginning to affect work then it is rea-sonable for a supervisor or appraiser to offer help and advice.

Domestic or financial problems at home may be causing a doctor great concern. Sometimes speaking to a supervisor or mentor about a situation helps an individual find a way forward. Some doctors need confidence to

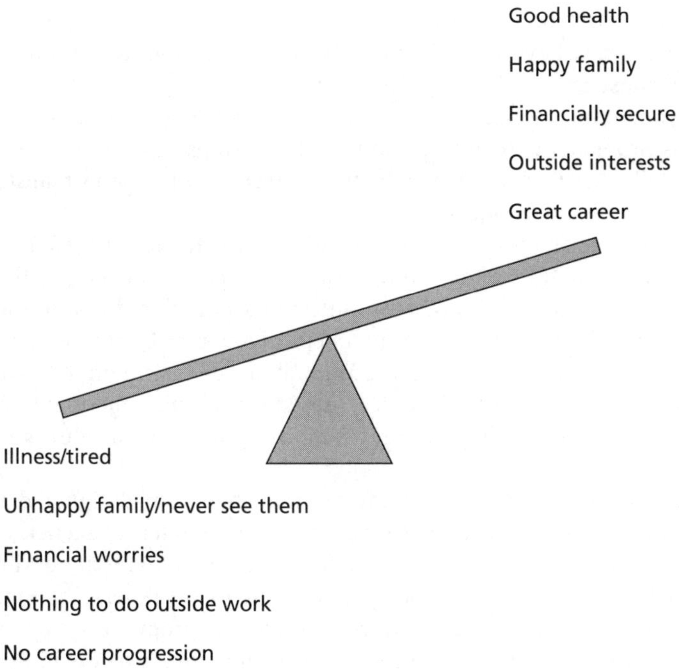

Good health

Happy family

Financially secure

Outside interests

Great career

Illness/tired

Unhappy family/never see them

Financial worries

Nothing to do outside work

No career progression

Figure 3.1 The work–life balance see-saw.

contact outside resources. Others might need encouragement to perhaps seek counselling. The most valuable resource is sometimes just having someone to speak to.

It may help to have job plans or timetables adjusted to help accommodate difficulties at home for a temporary period. There are very few jobs that are not amenable to flexibility. Often very small adjustments in a doctor's working day may help alleviate a difficult situation at home. Sometimes a period of annual leave or even unpaid leave can give the doctor time to resolve an issue at home that is affecting his or her performance at work.

Resources available to help doctors in difficulty

A number of different agencies have roles and responsibilities to help doctors in difficulty. Sometimes these overlap. Depending on the nature of the problem it is important to involve and seek assistance from the appropriate agency. The following is a brief description of the most important organisations and the assistance they can offer.

The deanery

The deanery should be the point of contact for any doctor in training who is experiencing difficulties. This can be done by the trainee, the educational supervisor or the training programme or foundation programme director. Many problems can be solved without involvement of the deanery but the postgraduate dean should always be informed about any ongoing significant issues.

Most deaneries have considerable resources available to help doctors in difficulty. These may include the following.

- Professional development programmes: these are regular courses that help address problems with interpersonal relationships and personal management skills. Many doctors benefit from meeting others and realising that their needs are not unique.
- One-to-one coaching: this may include preparing for the examination, developing language and communication skills and dealing with stress. Most deaneries will have access to outside coaching organisations and the coach can be identified to meet the needs of a particular trainee.
- Career counselling: an associate postgraduate dean is generally available for career counselling and advice, and in particular modified working arrangements such as less than full-time training, graded returns to work or career breaks.
- Confidential counselling: this may be available from designated trained individuals within the deanery or resourced from external agencies.

Advice on other issues such as immigration and employment conditions is also available. Initial contact should be with the medical personnel manager who can then point the doctor towards the most appropriate source of help. Many deaneries have specific protocols for dealing with doctors in difficulty, particularly with issues such as poor performance or conduct.

The deanery should be made aware of all significant conduct issues that arise for doctors in training. For serious acts of misconduct the deanery shares responsibility with the employer or trust for whom the doctor is working. If a doctor in training is the subject of suspension by the GMC or is subject to investigation, the deanery may also be able to offer advice and support for an eventual return to clinical practice.

The employer

The employer has overall responsibility for the conduct and performance of a doctor. It also has a responsibility to assist with work-based problems. Conduct problems should generally be referred via clinical directors to the medical director or a deputy with relevant responsibility. The employer will have a policy for instituting disciplinary action. This may involve suspension of the doctor from the workplace if this is deemed in the interests of patient safety.

Doctors with health issues may also be referred to occupational health by their employers and the employer has an obligation to assist with any changes to the workplace that may be necessary to help the doctor return to or continue in work. The employer also has a responsibility to assist with re-deployment if a doctor cannot continue his or her previous role.

The General Medical Council (GMC)

The GMC is the regulating body for all doctors. It deals with complaints and concerns that are reported by patients, doctors, employers, the police and other bodies. The GMC will take action if it feels that a doctor's fitness to practice is impaired. This may be because of misconduct, poor performance, a criminal conviction or caution and physical or mental ill health.

The GMC's procedures are divided into two stages: investigation and, when necessary, adjudication. The Interim Orders Panel can also suspend or place conditions on a doctor's registration. When a GMC investigation concludes that a doctor's fitness to practice is impaired, the GMC can suspend or remove a doctor from the medical register or place conditions on the doctor's registration. The GMC can also issue warnings to doctors when there has been a significant departure from the principles set out in its guidance for doctors, 'Good Medical Practice'.

The GMC aims to conduct its investigations as quickly as possible but a thorough investigation may take several months. During this time a doctor may require considerable support from supervisors or colleagues. The GMC will also appoint a named officer as a point of contact during an investigation and when there are health issues for the doctor concerned, a medical supervisor.

National Clinical Assessment Service (NCAS)

The NCAS promotes public confidence in doctors and dentists by helping to address concerns about individual practitioners. It also provides a confidential support service for doctors whose health is giving cause for concern. The NCAS may be contacted by the employer or the doctor him or herself.

The NCAS carries out assessments on practitioners in order to identify why the doctor is experiencing problems and what can be done to help. The NCAS advisors are drawn from a team of senior practitioners and managers based across the UK. They all have considerable experience in handling performance concerns. They provide telephone or face-to-face advice for local handling of concerns. They aim to work with all parties to clarify the concerns and make recommendations to help the practitioner continue to deliver high-quality, safe care for patients.

Defence organisations

Both the Medical Protection Society and the Medical Defence Union will support and assist doctors who experience difficulties at work and find themselves the subject of disciplinary action by an employer or investigation by the GMC. A key worker will be assigned to the case and advice will be provided by trained legal assessors. Key workers and legal professionals may also accompany doctors to hearings, case conferences and, when necessary, court attendances.

The British Medical Association (BMA)

The BMA will provide members with advice on contractual and workplace issues. They may also offer advice and support to doctors who are being investigated by the GMC. Like the defence organisations, they may also offer representatives who can support doctors and advise at case conferences and disciplinary hearings. They also offer a confidential counselling service to their members.

Summary

Helping doctors in difficulty can be a challenging but rewarding process for those involved. A supportive but fair approach is vital, as is a good knowledge of the resources available to help. Recognition of the problem, good documentation and clear communication with an agreed action plan are the four essential components of managing a doctor in difficulty.

Life consists not in holding good cards but in playing those you hold well.
J. BILLINGS

Bibliography

1. Department of Health. Maintaining high professional standards in the modern NHS. A framework for the initial handling of concerns about doctors and dentists in the NHS. DH, London, 2003. URL http://www.dh.gov.uk/en/Publicationsandsta tistics/Publications/PublicationsPolicyAndGuidance/DH_4072773

2. National Clinical Assessment Service handbook, 4th edition. URL http://www. ncas.npsa.nhs.uk/EasySiteWeb/GatewayLink.aspx?alId=10651
3. General Medical Council. Raising concerns about patient safety. GMC, London. URL http://www.gmc-uk.org/guidance/current/library/raising_concerns.asp
4. General Medical Council. A guide for doctors reported to the GMC. GMC, London. URL   http://www.gmc-uk.org/concerns/doctors_under_investigation/guide_for_ doctors.pdf
5. Department of Health. Mental health and employment in the NHS. DH, London, 2002. URL http://www.dh.gov.uk/en/Publicationsandstatistics/Publications/Public ationsPolicyAndGuidance/DH_4008361
6. A guide to postgraduate specialty training in the UK (The gold guide) (2007) URL http://www.mmc.nhs.uk/Docs/A%20Guide%20to%20Postgraduate%20Specialty %20Training%20in%20the%20UK%20(Gold%20Guide).doc

Further resources

• National Association of Clinical Tutors. Managing trainees in difficulty. Practical advice for educational and clinical supervisors. NACT, 2008. http://nact.org.uk/did.html
• Cox J, King J, Hutchinson A, McAvoy P. Understanding doctors' performance. Radcliffe Publishing, Oxford, 2005.
• A comprehensive list of all general and specialist services for doctors, both regional and national, can be found on the BMA website at: http://www.bma.org.uk/.

Key services include

1. BMA Counselling Service. Provides 24 hour telephone support by British Association of Counselling and Psychotherapy (BACP) accredited counsellors. Tel.: 08459 200169.
2. BMA Doctors for Doctors Service (DfD). DfD is an enhancement of the BMA Counselling Service giving doctors in distress or difficulty the choice of speaking in confidence to another doctor. The service is confidential and is not linked to any other external or internal agencies. Tel.: 020 7383 6739 or email: dfd@bma.org.uk (telephone and face-to-face appointments available).
3. Doctors' Support Network. Self-help group for doctors with mental health problems, website: www.dsn.org.uk
4. Royal Medical Benevolent Fund. Provides financial help for sick doctors. Tel.: 020 8540 9194, email: seniorcaseworker@rmbf.org, website: www.rmbf.org
5. Sick Doctors' Trust. A pro-active, self-help organisation for addicted physicians. Tel. (24 hour helpline): 0870 444 5163, website: www.sick-doctors-trust.co.uk
6. MedNet provides doctors and dentists working in the area covered by the London deanery with practical advice about their career, emotional support should they need it and, if appropriate, access to brief or longer term psychotherapy. The service operates on a strictly confidential basis. Tel.: 020 8938 2411, website: www.londondeanery.ac.uk/MedNet/

CHAPTER 4

Career planning and advice

Jane V. Howard[1] & David Clegg[2]
[1]The West Yorkshire Foundation School, Leeds, UK
[2]University of Leeds, Leeds, UK

Support for effective career planning is an integral part of training in modern postgraduate medicine. Ideally, career planning should start in medical school, but the transition from student to working doctor often requires a re-evaluation of plans as specialties come to be viewed in a different light. Training programmes can be designed to enable new medical graduates to explore a range of career opportunities in different areas of medicine. While there are many advantages of current structured training programmes, it does mean that applicants for higher specialist training tend to have had very similar experiences, and standing out from the crowd is more challenging. There is pressure on trainees to make career decisions earlier in their training so that their applications are appropriately focussed and there is also pressure to get the decision right first time, to avoid the difficulties in changing specialty later.

The need for career planning and advice

The National Institute for Careers Education and Counselling (NICEC) conducted a large survey of medical trainees in 2003. It found a high level of dissatisfaction with careers advice and planning, and concluded [1]:

> That a proactive and educational approach to career advice and guidance provision is required. Medical career advice and guidance should be positioned as part of medical training, and making sure that doctors have the opportunity to acquire the skills to manage their careers should be an integral part of that training. This implies a fundamental change of mindset in the whole approach to career advice and guidance for medical students and doctors in training. Equipping doctors to manage their own careers requires the development of interventions to enable individuals to:
> • develop career management skills;

Essential Guide to Educational Supervision in Postgraduate Medical Education.
Edited by Nicola Cooper and Kirsty Forrest. © 2009 Blackwell Publishing,
ISBN: 978-1-4051-7071-0.

- understand their interests and appraise their strengths and weaknesses;
- develop action plans for their career development and make more informed career decisions.

Box 4.1 gives a summary of the NICEC report's arguments and the changes recommended in the medical career advice arena. Its findings demonstrated that doctors have real problems deciding on their career and training choices [1]: 'It is wasteful and ineffective to keep ignoring this problem when a proactive and educational approach to career advice and guidance could make the complex career choice process less painful and more effective. More informed career choices by medical students and doctors in training would offer multiple benefits. Waiting until doctors encounter career problems is costly both to the individuals involved and the health care system in this country'.

Box 4.1 Results of the NICEC survey

Arguments for change:
1. The wider issue of medical morale
Many doctors in training managed their careers in spite of the system rather than with any active support. They frequently felt they could have made better career decisions. They wanted more active support for career decision-making than they received. The kinds of support advocated below would not be expensive compared with the costs of medical training and could generate significant benefits in terms of morale.
2. The dependence of the NHS on large numbers of overseas doctors
The survey provides evidence that overseas doctors feel marginalised, and that they also have additional advice and guidance needs. A more diverse medical workforce will have even greater need for career advice and guidance to ensure that medical careers are pursued on a level playing field.
3. The persistent problems of combining medical training with family life
These are aggravating shortages in certain specialties, distorting the deployment of the increasing number of female doctors and potentially undermining the general future supply of students willing to study medicine. Although improved career advice and guidance will not solve the problem of work–life balance in medical careers, it will help people prepare for and cope with it.
4. Deployment of skills
Doctors are very expensive to train and it is important that they find their way into areas of medicine that they are good at, as well as ones they like. In other organisations with highly skilled workforces, the deployment and development of scarce skills is the main driver for

---

(*Continued*)

> **Box 4.1** (Continued)
>
> paying attention to career choice and investing in improved career advice.
>
> Summary of the changes recommended:
> * A new role for careers education
> * Improved career information
> * Development of self-assessment and planning tools
> * Trained career contacts and improved support networks
> * Availability of impartial and expert advice
> * National co-ordination

Doctors' expectations of their career are changing and many no longer assume they will stay in the same job throughout their lives. They may wish to diversify into other aspects of medicine, for example management or education, or focus on developing more specialised clinical interests and skills. They may also move to a career outside medicine. Many issues can drive this: personal circumstances, interests, work–life balance problems and burnout. Similarly, health system expectations are changing and doctors have an increasing contribution to management, development of health services, education and training.

No one can make a doctor's career decisions for him or her, but as an educational supervisor you can help and support your trainees in their decision. Even if career planning were not a formal part of your role, it is likely that trainees would still come to you for advice. The General Medical Council's (GMC) survey of UK graduate doctors in 2006 showed that 88% of trainees sought career advice from senior colleagues in their organisation [2]. Clearly the demand is there, and an expectation that there will be constructive and realistic support for career planning. Other people are also able to offer career support. Box 4.2 shows the key people that can be involved.

> **Box 4.2**
>
> Key people who can help with career planning:
> * Deanery careers advisers
> * Training programme directors
> * College tutors/regional specialty advisers
> * Regional educational advisers
> * Friends and colleagues
> * Educational supervisors
> * University careers advisers
> * National Health Service employment advice centres

The rest of this chapter will outline the principles of career planning and examples of practical steps for delivering individual and group careers advice and guidance. While helping your trainees, you may find that being involved in delivering careers advice also provides you with an opportunity to objectively review your own career and future.

Principles of effective career planning and advice

The *Operational Framework for Foundation Programmes* [3] defines career planning as: 'doctors learning and being coached about how best to match their skills, strengths and interests with the needs of the NHS'. It is likely that this principle will underpin any future career framework for all postgraduate doctors.

This process of matching self-awareness (one's skills, strengths and interests) to opportunities (the needs of the NHS) fits in with the 'DOTS model' of career management [4]. See Box 4.3.

Box 4.3

The 'DOTS model' of career management:
Decision learning
• Learning decision-making styles and making career decisions
Opportunity awareness
• Knowing what opportunities are out there
• Knowing what they require and what they have to offer
Transition learning
• Making the transition from where you are now to where you want to be
• Action planning and application strategies
Self-awareness
• Knowing what you have to offer and what you want from a career

---

In 2005, the Modernising Medical Careers (MMC) working group for career management published *Career Management: An Approach for Medical Schools, Deaneries, Royal Colleges and Trusts* [5]. The report included 14 proposed initiatives, listed in Box 4.4 with examples, to support the career planning of doctors and medical students. Although it is not a formal policy, the document provides a useful starting point to help review the support currently in place and to develop new initiatives.

The following section will give specific examples of support for individual career planning within a region or institution. These examples have been developed locally and are evolving. All examples are used as an illustration, with the readers free to take and use what will help in their own context.

Box 4.4 Proposed initiatives

1. *Career information sources*
   - Develop a careers website with regional/local specialty information and links to other web-based medical careers information sources (e.g. NHS careers, MMC).
   - Include careers information in your hospital education centre library
   - Liaise with your University Careers Service who will have a wide range of resources covering general medical and related healthcare careers alongside material covering non-medical careers.
2. *Career conference*
   - Career conferences or careers fairs allow trainees to hear about a range of career options and to speak to consultants and royal college representatives.
   - Involving medical students and foundation doctors in the development and organisation of careers fairs allows them to develop and demonstrate key skills in areas such as organisation, communication and negotiation, and helps to ensure relevant content.
   - Holding events covering specific specialty areas, for example a 'careers in surgery day' with speakers and exhibition stands from sub-specialties within that discipline, also helps.
3. *Career forums*
   - Hold smaller events comprising presentations and discussions around a particular specialty. These could be developed and delivered by groups of students and trainees.
4. *Career handbook/resource*
   - A published resource including information on career options, useful advice, specialty information etc.
5. *Online guidance discussions*
   - These can be website discussion boards or simpler email services.
   - University Careers Centres often have email services, and Prospects Web offers a national email service for graduates.
6. *Peer group activities*
   - Groups of foundation doctors could work together to deliver careers information sessions to colleagues, to develop other peer support activities around career planning, and to prepare for the applications process and interviews.
7. *Specialist career planning tools/programmes*
   - Sci59 is a specialty choice inventory available online: http://sci59.open.ac.uk/sci59public/index.php
   - Prospects Planner covers graduate level recruitment and will be of interest to doctors considering options outside medicine: www.prospects.ac.uk/links/Pplanner/

(Continued)

Box 4.4 (Continued)

- Trainees should not be encouraged to use these tools in isolation; discussing the results and reflecting on the process is vital and often more useful than simply looking at the top entries on the results page.

8. *Focussed experiences*
   - Specialty tasters are vital to give trainees the opportunity to experience specialties that may not feature in their training programme.

9. *Designated careers advisers*
   - Your deanery may have appointed a careers adviser who is able to offer individual careers advice to doctors.
   - You will be able to refer doctors for support, or help promote the services offered by the careers adviser so doctors can self-refer as appropriate.

10. *Designated trained career contacts*
    - Most deaneries will offer careers guidance skills courses for senior registrars and consultants. These courses ensure trainees have access to appropriate and consistent careers support at a local level.

11. *Medical school support services*
    - Medical schools and university careers services provide a wide range of services to facilitate and support effective career management.
    - Other partners such as counselling services also offer complimentary services – although not focussed on careers, they may deal with issues that impact on an individual's career management, decision-making and future plans.

12. *Postgraduate deanery guidance and support services*
    - Deaneries have a range of support services to help doctors, including individual support provided by associate deans (e.g. careers and personal development, foundation programmes and overseas doctors), educational advisers and careers advisers.
    - Relevant information should be available on deanery websites that outline how you can access these resources and refer doctors for support.

Individual career support

The main aim of support with career planning is to help your trainees progress:
- in their decision-making;
- with their application strategies;
- from where they are now to where they want to be.

Individual career advice or guidance is an important element of career planning for trainee doctors and may take the form of a formal interview, brief discussion as part of an appraisal or review meeting or ad hoc conversations. Whatever the location and duration, it is possible to deliver effective advice by following a well-established career guidance model; this will help focus the conversation and ensure you work towards clear action points to help your trainees move on.

Career interviews can be broadly categorised into four main areas:

- *Information*
  Factual information about a specialty, other career opportunities and the application process.
- *Advice*
  An immediate response to the needs of a trainee who presents an enquiry or reveals a need that requires more than straightforward information, for example interpreting information or applying it to his or her own circumstances.
- *Guidance*
  A more in-depth interview that helps trainees to explore a range of options, to analyse and relate information to their own needs and circumstances and to make decisions about their careers. Effective career guidance should be non-directive and trainee-centred, working to help them come up with the answers and plans for their next steps.
- *Counselling*
  'Counselling takes place when a counsellor sees a client in a private and confidential setting to explore a difficulty the client is having, distress they may be experiencing or perhaps their dissatisfaction with life, or loss of a sense of direction and purpose' [6]. If you feel a trainee does require counselling you will have to consider whether the best response would be to refer to a more appropriate support, for example an independent counselling service, rather than try to offer counselling within a career interview. Often, if there are wider issues around depression or anxiety, these need to be addressed before effective career guidance and career planning can take place.

It is neither always easy to clearly see what a trainee is seeking, nor possible to define a particular interview as either 'information' or 'guidance'. The categories listed above often overlap, as illustrated in Box 4.5.

Overlap may arise from the trainees presenting requests for information as a means of establishing the relationship, waiting until they feel more comfortable or confident with the support you are offering before disclosing deeper statements and concerns that require guidance. You may choose to move an information request into the guidance realm; for example, if trainees approach with an information request, you can move the discussion into guidance by asking how they decided which specialty to apply for, what research they have done into how their skills and qualities relate to their chosen specialty, and how they have reflected on their experiences to identify examples to use in their application form or interview.

Box 4.5

The overlap between different types of career advice meetings

Information/advice	Advice/guidance	Guidance/counselling
How do I get into cardiology?	I'm not sure which specialty is right for me.	I'm really distressed and demoralised by the whole system.
What selection process will I go through to get on to GP training?	I'm not getting shortlisted.	I want to leave medicine, what other careers are open to me?
Where are the vacancies advertised?	I'm regularly invited to interview, but haven't had any job offers.	I find it a real struggle to get myself into work.
How many jobs are there in paediatrics in this deanery?	I'm not really sure which specialty I'd enjoy.	I don't think I ever really wanted to get into medicine and I've started to wish I'd done a different degree.
Whom should I consult to find out more about a career in sports medicine?	Which specialty do you think I should apply for?	I'm on medication for depression and my job has contributed to my illness.

Managing an effective career interview

A common approach to effective career guidance interviews is the counselling approach of Ali and Graham [7]. Do not let the title deceive you into thinking this is about delivering counselling; it is not. It is, however, about using the trainee-centred, non-directive approach of counselling to help structure career interviews effectively.

The model defines the careers interview in four stages and can be applied to a five-minute discussion in the coffee room or a formal forty-five-minute guidance interview.

- *Clarifying*
  Here you set the scene, listen to initial questions and comments and start to make an assessment about how to approach the interview.
- *Exploring*
  This is where you build the contract and start to explore the main issues put forward by the trainee, whilst also encouraging him or her to explore other options.
- *Evaluating*
  Here you will help the trainee to evaluate the options (e.g. looking at pros and cons), challenge any inconsistencies and look at the trainee's priorities.

- *Action planning*
  Your trainee needs to own the action plan, but you can help him or her
  identify key tasks that need to be done and when they need to be done.

You can see how this interview structure fits with the 'DOTS model' – the
clarifying and exploring stages allow exploration of self-awareness and opportunity awareness; in the evaluating phase, the trainees start exploring the
options open to them and making effective decisions; and in the action planning stage, they plan how they can make the transition to their next post. This
may not all take place in one interview, for example if a doctor has low levels
of self-awareness the outcome and action plan might be more about developing in these areas rather than putting an application together; however, overall
it is useful to keep both models in mind when undertaking career interviews.

Specialty tasters

Embedded taster programmes are a feature of the foundation curriculum
and a suggested way to utilise available study leave. The objectives are to
gauge whether personal attributes and skills suit the workload and case mix,
and to appreciate life as a specialist, particularly the differences between junior and senior roles.

Specialty tasters also serve to demonstrate a commitment to the specialty
and find out what sort of people it attracts. In practical terms, one- or two-day
attachments in up to three different specialties are encouraged. A taster direc-
tory with names and contact details for all the specialties is provided locally.
The trainees are encouraged to talk to anyone and everyone who might have
something useful to say about their abilities, personality and what it takes to
have a healthy career in the specialty they are considering. Trainees are asked
to keep a specialty taster review form as part of their portfolio, the essential
components of which are given in Box 4.6. This form can help provide evidence and information for discussion in applications and interviews.

Box 4.6 Specialty taster review form

- What is the key information about this specialty that you gathered
  from this experience?
- Which skills are vital for work in this specialty?
- What are the positive and negative elements to a career in this
  specialty?
- Would you be interested in pursuing a career in this specialty?
- If 'yes' or 'don't know', what could you do to find out more to make
  sure this is the right decision and improve your chances of selection?
- If 'no', why not? How might this experience be useful for your appli-
  cation to other specialties?
- Have your views about this specialty changed after this experience?

Supporting doctors seeking careers outside medicine

Doctors may be looking at options outside medicine for a number of reasons.

- As a choice – they realise that medicine is not right for them.
- As advised – there is hardly any progress through their training.
- As an alternative to unemployment – they are not being appointed to the deanery or specialty of their choice.

This can be a very stressful time for the individual concerned, especially if there is a real prospect of unemployment. It can also be stressful for the educational supervisor trying to give advice. You cannot be expected to be an expert in non-medical careers, and there are an increasing number of resources to which you can refer trainees for more appropriate information and advice.

- Prospects: www.prospects.ac.uk is the UK's official graduate careers website and includes 'Prospects Planner', an interactive careers tool.
- Doctor Job: www.doctorjob.com is a website from Group GTI (www.targetjobs.co.uk), a large publisher of graduate careers information.
- Graduate Employment and Training: www.get.hobsons.co.uk is the website that can be accessed.

The trainees may also be able to access the local university career service for advice and information on non-medical options. Universities have different policies for dealing with graduate work – some will only see their own graduates, some will see graduates from anywhere, and some may be part of regionally co-ordinated projects.

Pastoral support can be invaluable in this situation, and services such as Support4Doctors (www.support4doctors.org) can be useful sources of support, especially if the move out of medicine is driven by external factors rather than the trainee's own career plans.

Group career support

There are obvious advantages in providing career guidance to a group (e.g. time and cost); however, there is also the social advantage of group support and sharing knowledge. Private companies exist which provide training packages with facilitators who will deliver sessions in your institution. For example, Windmills™ is based on a partnership between the University of Liverpool, Graduate into Employment Unit and Dr Peter Hawkins, and has delivered this type of training across the UK [8].

Some regions, such as our own, have developed their own training programmes. Career support has been embedded into our local compulsory professional development programme (PDP) for foundation trainees and developed further for specialist trainees. A day-long session is delivered in a variety of ways depending on the local circumstances. These are supplemented with lunchtime teaching sessions, a work book and a website, to ensure all trainees have access to the same support material and exercises.

The sessions are run in tutorial style with small groups. This means sessions need to be repeated across the region and rely on goodwill and help of clinical colleagues. Facilitators are recruited from educational supervisors, training programme directors, and college tutors. Senior registrars may also be keen to help as facilitators.

Given the potentially sensitive nature of some of the discussions, a supportive atmosphere is fostered within the group. Rather than having a list of strict rules to follow, the discussion is around the need for respect, sensitivity and confidentiality throughout the session. This can also be linked to professionalism, which is useful as it features on person specifications.

The first half of the programme focuses on self-awareness, opportunity awareness and decision-making. Being clear about key skills, interests and work values helps trainees decide for what and where they are going to apply, and also provides data for any written applications, curriculum vitae and interview material. The second half of the programme focuses on transition, with the aim of providing practical support for applications. Box 4.7 has an overview of an example programme.

The content of the session is based loosely on the 'DOTS model'. This model appears more logical when seen in a different order; understanding of self and the opportunities available allows one to make a decision and put a plan into action, aiming towards a positive transition as seen in Figure 4.1.

Box 4.7 Overview of an example programme

0830	Coffee and registration
0845	Welcome, introductions and ground rules
0900	Specialty options
1000	Specialty training person specifications and identifying generic skills
1030	Break
1045	Medical skills
1130	Making yourself more competitive
1150	Summary
1200	Lunch
1300	Effective applications presentation
1330	Applications exercise
1415	Short listing group exercise
1500	Break
1515	Applications and group feedback
1530	Interviews presentation
1545	Interviews exercise

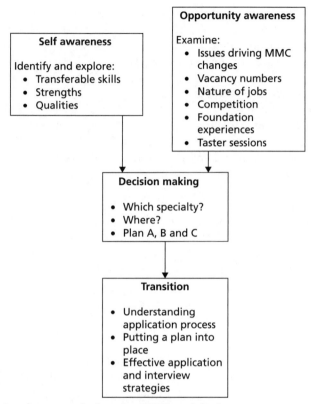

Figure 4.1 Another way to look at the 'DOTS model' of career management.

Specialty options

Reasons for speciality choices are explored. Analysing competition ratios to look at which specialties have most vacancies, how competitive they are and what the training pathways are like, including the options available after core training, is a key feature of choosing a speciality. To prompt initial large-group discussion, or for contemplation in smaller groups, two questions are posed.

- Are skills, strengths and interests the only factors that influence your choice of career? If not, what else do you need to consider?
- What are the needs of the National Health Service (NHS)?

The first question stimulates lively discussion about other factors driving the career decision-making process. Not surprisingly, there are many factors beyond their own 'skills, strengths and interests' that are important when choosing a career. As for the needs of the NHS, this usually provides interesting debate and comment. The kind of responses given in our sessions are listed in Box 4.8.

Previous research looking at the attractiveness of medical careers does back up our local findings. After factors such as clinical freedom, team-working,

Box 4.8

Responses to the questions:

Are skills, strengths and interests the only factors that influence your choice of career?

If not, what else do you need to consider?
- Pay and conditions
- Geography – not just at deanery level but where you end up actually working
- Enjoyment (and do you enjoy it enough to relocate?)
- Quality of life and a good work–life balance
- The demands of the job/specialty
- Competition
- Prospects and future opportunities
- Flexible training and availability of part-time work
- Family and lifestyle
- On-call responsibilities
- Job security
- Holidays

What are the needs of the NHS?
- Cheap labour
- Commitment
- Loyalty
- Service provision
- A certain number of doctors in a certain number of places
- More doctors and better doctors
- As few doctors as possible
- More consultants
- Less consultants

variation in tasks and continuity of care, the next four most important factors are flexible working, control over working patterns, personal time and family life. The three most common factors identified as unattractive in a career are management work, professional isolation and paperwork [9].

When making the decision on which speciality to enter, the person specifications for each speciality are useful to look at. The MMC website contains a comprehensive list of person specifications for specialist training appointments, divided into 12 categories (see Box 4.9); each category in turn has further requirements [10].

Two exercises are used to look at the generic skills from the speciality person specifications to raise trainees' self-awareness in these areas. These exercises help them focus on how they can support their applications within their portfolios, during the application process and at the time of interview.

Box 4.9 Person specification headings for specialist training appointments

- Qualifications
- Eligibility
- Fitness to practice
- Language skills
- Health
- Career progression
- Application completion
- Clinical skills
- Academic and research skills
- Personal skills
- Probity
- Commitment to specialty

From www.mmc.nhs.uk

Non-medical examples

The trainees are asked to select a skill from interests and activities outside work. This is encouraged to demonstrate the importance of reflecting on skills and being able to transfer and relate these abilities to different situations. The group divides into pairs with each member of the pair choosing one of these skills for their partner to write about. We use a proforma with the following four headings.

- Skill: This refers to whichever skill they are writing about from the list.
- Example or activity: This refers to a description of where and how they used this skill.
- Evidence: This refers to the documentation or other evidence they have that might be included in their portfolio.
- Relevance to chosen specialty: This relates how this experience and skill is relevant to the specialty to which they are applying.

An example might be playing a sport or a musical instrument that can be reflected upon as team-work or manual dexterity, and how that might be useful for a career in general practice or surgery.

Medical examples

Written examples of the different skills relevant to each specialty from a number of person specifications are distributed randomly among the pairs. They then use the same proforma as before. After working through this in pairs, it is useful to get the whole group to talk about the examples they used, how they could see the relevance to their chosen specialties, how easy or difficult they found it, and whether they felt prepared to discuss these areas in an application form or interview. In addition, this can help focus the trainees' minds on what they think they are good at and enjoy doing.

Having explored some of the influences on career choice, our next step is to identify where the trainees are now with respect to career planning, under the following headings.

- I have chosen the specialty I wish to pursue.
- I am not certain which specialty I wish to pursue, but I have started to narrow it down.
- I have not yet decided which specialty I wish to pursue, and I have not yet started to narrow it down.

Question sheets (see Box 4.10) with different questions aimed at each group are given to the trainees and they are allocated 15 min to work through them individually.

Box 4.10

Where am I now?

I have chosen the specialty I wish to pursue.	I am not certain but I have started to narrow it down.	I have not yet decided or narrowed it down.
How did you make this decision?	Specialties I am considering are:	What are you looking for in a specialty or career?
What have you done to be certain this is the right choice?	Specialties I have definitely ruled out are:	What are your key skills and qualities you wish to use in your work?
What skills and qualities do you have to make you a good candidate?	What is it about the specialties you are considering that makes them attractive to you?	What are your values and interests that motivate you?
What are the main attractions or features of the specialty that make it right for you?	What do you need to do to start narrowing your choices down and come to a decision?	What can you do to start narrowing down your choices and making decisions?
What do you know about how competitive opportunities in this specialty will be?	How will you know if you have made the right decision?	

These questions are very similar to those found on application forms. They are very likely to come up at the time of interview, and can demonstrate that trainees have the motivations, skills and insight to be successful in their chosen specialty.

Becoming more competitive

This session starts to draw conclusions from the earlier ones and discusses strategies for becoming more competitive. The emphasis during the discussion develops along the following lines:

- considering career opportunities carefully;
- understanding the transferable nature of one's skills;
- making the most of current opportunities;
- networking to identify new opportunities;
- being inventive and original;
- getting it all documented for one's portfolio.

Evidence gathered from the above exercises is linked with personal reviews from their posts and taster sessions so far. The next step is transition skills to help them make a positive move from where they are now to where they want to be. Although they may have encountered structured application forms before, they may not be comfortable or confident in answering them. Not all foundation schools use interviews as part of the selection process, so for many trainees their core training interviews may be their first serious interview.

Effective applications

One of the relatively new aspects of postgraduate medical applications is the notorious 'white space' boxes that need to be filled in. Useful strategies and models are presented to trainees to help them with this task. One model that applies to application forms and interviews (and, to a lesser extent, curriculum vitae) is the StAR model:

- *Situation or task*
  The introduction, outlining the situation or task they were faced with.
- *Action or activities*
  The bulk of the answer, what they actually did, clearly showing their role, contribution, skills and qualities.
- *Result or reflection*
  A quick summary of the results of their actions (ideally positive). This can also show reflection on performance and situations.

This model is encouraged in the following exercises.

Applications exercise

A mini application form of three questions with a 150-word limit per answer is given to the trainees, who have 30 min to complete two questions. These are real questions from previous anonymous foundation or specialty training application forms. This part of the day leads to much discussion about creative writing, but the end-of-day evaluations reveal that trainees find this the most useful exercise. Box 4.11 has examples of some of the questions.

Box 4.11 Examples of the questions for the application process

- Give an example of a non-academic achievement, explaining both the significance to you and the relevance to your medical training.
- Describe an example of a situation in which you had to demonstrate your professionalism and/or integrity. What did you do and what was the outcome?
- Describe an example from your own experience that has increased your understanding of team-working. What was your role and contribution?

Short listing group exercise

The group is then divided into short listing panels. Each panel is given a small number of application forms to mark, making sure that none of the applications were written by the group members. The forms are anonymous, but coded so that individuals can receive feedback at the end of the day if they wish. The panel is asked to work together to shortlist the top 50% of forms and provide a summary of key positive and negative feedback points to be shared with the whole group.

This kind of activity works really well as trainees get a chance to see real forms, grasp what works and what does not, and see how easy it is to make positive and negative impressions. The feedback they give and receive reinforces the learning points, helping them to start their preparation for the real process. Some key points raised by our groups are summarised in Box 4.12.

Box 4.12 Key learning points raised from the discussion on short listing written applications

- Penalties for those not following instructions became obvious.
- The relevance of examples or scenarios written in answer to a question was not always clear.
- Recent scenarios are better than older examples.
- Legibility and grammar, spelling and avoidance of abbreviations are important.
- Language is important in creating a positive impression.
- There are difficulties in not sounding 'corny'.
- Simple was often more effective.
- Trying to give people the benefit of the doubt was sometimes very difficult.

One of the key feedback areas is always spelling and grammar. This reminds us of the applicant who claimed to be 'gaol [*sic*] oriented' or the one who wrote 'excellent communications kills'.

Interviews

The session finishes with interview work, with a presentation on effective interview technique covering important areas.

- Body language
- Irrelevant answers
- Badly organised answers
- Recited answers
- Repetition
- Nervousness or lack of confidence
- Overconfidence
- A very quick or very slow mode of conversation
- Failure to engage the entire panel

This is followed by mock interviews with each trainee playing the role of a candidate interviewed by a panel of their colleagues. Lists of example questions are given, or trainees can select their own questions from earlier real-life experiences. Easier questions like, 'Why this speciality?' are a good place to start. This session also gives an opportunity to explore strategies for dealing with unusual questions such as, 'If you could describe yourself as an animal which would it be and why?' It also gives the opportunity to reflect on interview gaffes such as the Emergency Medicine applicant who asked at the end of the interview, 'Do I have to work Friday nights?', or the candidate who when asked, 'How many hours a week can a doctor work under European Working Time Directive?' responded, 'Eighteen'.

More and more interviews are including team exercises, simulated patient consultations, written exercises and Objective Structured Clinical Examinations (OSCEs). We will endeavour to replicate some of these in our sessions in the future.

Summary

Choosing a career can be stressful, compounded by the common misconception that there is a single right answer and getting it wrong can be disastrous. This is simply not true. Doctors are intelligent, committed and competent people who can make a success of almost anything they turn their hand to.

Implementing some of the activities outlined in this chapter and adopting a proactive approach to supporting your trainees' career planning can help them make effective career decisions, help with their applications and make them respond quickly and positively to any subsequent change and uncertainty they may face during their career.

Finally, career advice should not stop in the early years of postgraduate training. It is essential to provide information about opportunities for further career development and even make positive plans for changes until retirement.

References

1. Jackson C, Ball J, Hirsh W, Kidd JM. National Institute for Careers Education and Counselling (NICEC). Informing choices: the need for career advice in medical training. NICEC, London, 2003. www.crac.org.uk/crac_new/pdfs/informingchoices_medicaltraining.pdf
2. General Medical Council. Survey of UK graduate doctors. GMC, London, 2006. www.gmc-uk.org/doctors/documents
3. Modernising Medical Careers. Operational framework for the Foundation programme, 2007. www.foundationprogramme.nhs.uk
4. Law B, Watts AG. Schools, careers and community. Church Information Office, London, 1977.
5. Modernising Medical Careers Working Group for Career Management. Career management: an approach for Medical Schools, Deaneries, Royal Colleges and Trusts. MMC, London, 2005.
6. British Association of Counselling and Psychotherapy. What is counselling? www.bacp.co.uk/education/whatiscounselling.html
7. Ali L, Graham B. The counselling approach to careers guidance. Routledge, London, 1996.
8. www.windmillsonline.co.uk, The Windmills™ website.
9. Blades DS, Ferguson G, Richardson HC, Redfern N. A study of junior doctors to investigate the factors that influence career decisions. *Br J Gen Pract* 2000; **50 (455)**: 483–485.
10. Person specifications. www.mmc.nhs.uk

Further resources

• BMJ careers advice online – http://careers.bmj.com/careers/advice
• British Medical Association. Sign-posting medical careers for doctors. www.bma.org.uk/ap.nsf/Content/signposting
• www.nhscareers.nhs.uk
• Chambers R, Mohanna K, Thornett A, Field S. Guiding doctors in managing their careers: a toolkit for tutors, trainers, mentors and appraisers. Radcliffe, Oxford, 2006.

CHAPTER 5

Putting a curriculum into practice

Nicola Cooper[1] & Colin R. Melville[2]
[1]The Leeds Teaching Hospitals NHS Trust, Leeds, UK
[2]North Yorkshire East Coast Foundation School; Hull York Medical School; Hull and East Yorkshire NHS Trust, Hull, UK

This chapter describes some of the issues involved in putting a curriculum into practice. It focuses on the 'big picture': what a curriculum is, the role of educational supervisors and trainees and a variety of examples that demonstrate how some aspects of specialty curricula have been put into practice. The next chapter discusses teaching and learning at a more individual level, including the development of professional expert practice.

What is a curriculum?

The word 'curriculum' has its origins in the running tracks and chariot courses of Ancient Greece and derives from the Latin word *currere* that means 'to run'. The Postgraduate Medical Education and Training Board (PMETB) defines a curriculum as: 'a statement of the intended aims and objectives, content, experiences, outcomes and processes of an educational programme including:
- a description of the training structure (entry requirements, length and organisation of the programme including its flexibilities, and assessment system) and
- a description of expected methods of learning, teaching, feedback and supervision' [1].

A curriculum is therefore everything that happens in relation to an educational programme. This includes its intentions, outcomes and processes (Figure 5.1). A curriculum is different from a syllabus, which is a list of knowledge, skills and attitudes to attain. So if there is a document that contains these elements then we have our curriculum ready to put into practice – well, not quite!

Essential Guide to Educational Supervision in Postgraduate Medical Education.
Edited by Nicola Cooper and Kirsty Forrest. © 2009 Blackwell Publishing,
ISBN: 978-1-4051-7071-0.

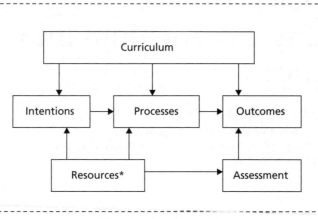

Figure 5.1 A network diagram of a curriculum showing intentions, processes and outcomes.
*Resources includes educational, people, time, information technology, financial etc.

A curriculum is more than a document, and the document is not the only curriculum that exists. For every formal curriculum there is the informal, the hidden and the assessed curricula. The formal curriculum consists of the curriculum on paper and, to some extent, the way it is put into practice. The informal curriculum includes what learners actually experience, and the hidden curriculum includes things that learners *infer* to be important. Ideally these should all overlap very closely, but they often do not (Figure 5.2). All curricula

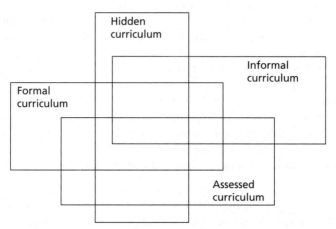

Figure 5.2 The formal, informal, hidden and assessed curricula. Ideally these should all overlap very closely.

take place in an educational environment, which in itself has an important impact on learning.

The informal, hidden and assessed curricula

The revised foundation programme curriculum, for example, emphasises that new doctors learn from practice in a clinical environment, rather than the classroom. It also stresses the concept of expertise, which is something different to competence, and is the goal of professional education. This concept is explored further in Chapter 6. However, as Fish and Coles point out, some of the language we use reveals a lack of understanding about education and professional education in particular. Some current misconceptions are as follows [2].

- Professional practice is a simple activity that yields to simple rules.
- Skills learning is about simple repetition.
- 'Competencies' = competence = performance.
- Competence is enough.
- Professional education and development requires professionals to leave their practice setting and [be taught] 'in protected time'.
- The quality of experience in postgraduate medical education is simply correlated to its amount.

There is a lot of evidence to suggest the opposite [3–6]. An informal curriculum may exist that emphasises these misconceptions rather than concepts that the formal curriculum tries to emphasise. An informal curriculum can arise from poor knowledge, skills and attitudes of faculty and trainees, or suboptimal organisation, content and quality of teaching and assessments. It has the potential to limit rather than enrich the education of doctors.

The hidden curriculum consists of the unwritten and unspoken factors in an educational programme. An important influence on learners is not necessarily what they are taught, but what they are modelled. For example, it has been shown that undergraduate medical students become demotivated by their perception that clinical teachers have a low level of commitment to teaching [7].

Davies illustrated one aspect of the hidden curriculum this way: 'the hidden curriculum can sometimes lurk behind the one we think we are teaching. The *way* we teach can sometimes contradict *what* we are teaching. We may think we are urging our students to become independent learners, critical thinkers and good clinical reasoners, using their adult maturity and experiences to take them beyond the textbook learning of their [previous] experiences. But, in fact, our teaching styles and educational strategies may be just as teacher-centred, textbook-based and implicitly authority dependent…as the most traditional teaching of the nineteenth century' [8].

The assessed curriculum can also be different. It is impossible to assess an entire curriculum, so assessments are chosen to sample a variety of domains across a curriculum at different times. However, as the saying goes, 'assessment drives learning', so if you want trainees to be able to know, do or behave a certain way – assess it. The opposite of this can also apply – if trainees know that one aspect of the curriculum is not going to be assessed, they are unlikely to pay as much attention to it.

The spiral curriculum

The spiral curriculum is the description given to the process whereby topics are revisited over time with increasing levels of difficulty, new applications or further practical experience. New learning is related to previous learning, with the advantage of challenge and increasing 'competence'. It is based on the constructivist or building block model of learning – that is, learning takes place by building individual conceptual frameworks that are added to or revised as new information comes along. To some extent, this is what happens naturally in medical education.

The foundation programme curriculum is an example of a curriculum that embraces this spiral curriculum concept, and in describing its design, states that, 'Foundation doctors are developing professionals who need to deepen and broaden their understanding and expertise by:
- revisiting clinical and professional practice, and studying at increasingly complex levels;
- practising with decreasing supervision;
- building on existing levels of understanding and
- recognising that levels of expertise generally increase with practice and reflection' [9].

However, sometimes what we see in practice does not reflect a spiral curriculum at all. To illustrate the concept of a spiral curriculum, Figure 5.3 shows what one would look like for communication skills, starting at medical school (year 1) and continuing throughout postgraduate medical education (year 6+).

The learning environment

The various curricula take place within a learning environment and this refers to the 'atmosphere' or 'climate' of an educational unit. The environment is known to have an important impact on learning and has been studied extensively in undergraduate medical education. Positive and negative features about the learning environment are shown in Box 5.1 [10]. Constructive feedback and the promotion of critical thinking are other important predictors of learner satisfaction [11].

The positive aspects of a learning environment focus on relationships and personal development, whereas the negative aspects include organisational problems in addition to those related to relationship and person development.

Similar conclusions have been reached in research in the workplace [12]. The positive aspects of the workplace involve good relationships and personal development, whereas negative aspects involve poor systems and processes. When people work in an environment with poor systems and processes, a great deal of job dissatisfaction results, but the opposite is not true. Good

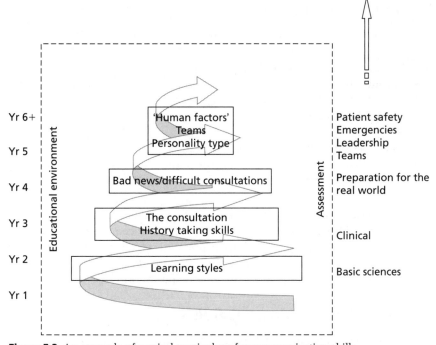

Figure 5.3 An example of a spiral curriculum for communication skills.
'Human factors' refers to the training in error, human performance and team
communication, which pilots have to undergo and is increasingly being applied to
healthcare.
Reproduced from Ref [25].

Box 5.1 Positive and negative features of the undergraduate learning
environment

Positive
• Relaxed atmosphere
• Encouragement of participation
• Enthusiasm of teachers
• Openness to discussion
• Good selection of patients
• Motivation
• Encouragement
• Adequate preparation

(*Continued*)

Box 5.1 (Continued)

Negative
- Conflicting information
- Late arrival/cutting tutorials short
- Missed tutorials
- Unreasonable expectations
- Patronising attitude
- Anger
- Victimisation of an individual
- Ridicule

systems and processes *alone* do not lead to job satisfaction. Something more is required in addition: responsibility, recognition, advancement and growth.

We can apply these principles to postgraduate medical education, where good systems relate to aspects such as clear and timely communication about posts, rotas, contracts, timetables, roles and expectations.

The role of educational supervisors

When it comes to putting a curriculum into practice, there are two main roles for educational supervisors. The first is to fully understand the formal curriculum, so that the informal and the hidden curricula do not predominate, as well as to contribute to a positive learning environment. The second is to give direction to trainees, so that they achieve the curriculum's aims and objectives for themselves.

The process of appraisal (discussed further in Chapter 8) provides one opportunity for educational supervisors to guide trainees on which elements of a curriculum can be achieved within a certain time frame, and which should be prioritised. If the model of the appraisal process is mapped to the Ancient Greek origins of the word, it provides for us the starting point (initial meeting), a check on the route being followed (mid-term review) and an end point (end of placement review).

The role of trainees

The trainees' role in their own education must not be forgotten. The foundation curriculum, for example, requires that trainees 'demonstrate the knowledge, attitudes, behaviours, skills and competencies needed to start self-directed life long learning', and describes key characteristics of learning in the clinical setting.
- It takes place during professional practice.
- It requires all clinical events to be seen and treated as educational experiences.

- Although carried out essentially in the practice setting, it must be complemented by opportunities for reflection (at a distance).

  The PMETB document, 'Standards for training for the Foundation Programme', states that, 'Foundation doctors have responsibilities which impact on the delivery of the curriculum, for example, providing feedback, participating in assessment and appraisal and completing the portfolio'. [13]

Therefore trainees have the following responsibilities when it comes to putting a curriculum into practice.

- They are required to adopt the knowledge, skills and attitudes of a self-directed learner.
- They should view clinical work as a learning opportunity.
- They should provide constructive feedback on the delivery of the curriculum.
- They should engage in work-based assessments as an educational exercise rather than a 'tick box' process. The assessment allows feedback on the teaching or curriculum delivery allied to that assessment and the opportunity to discuss further personal development.
- They are required to maintain a portfolio, including a personal development plan, which provides documentary evidence that the topics within the curriculum are being covered and that they have demonstrated 'competency' in each area.

All postgraduate medical curricula emphasise the need for trainees to be self-directed learners. Indeed, this does not just apply to trainees, but to doctors in general. Self-assessment is accepted as a prerequisite for continuing professional development. High-quality research in this area is scarce. However, a review of the available evidence on self-assessment identifies some key themes [14].

- Individuals can more accurately assess the performance of their peers than their own.
- Professionals must decide whether they have the competence to undertake a procedure, and this decision is based on their *confidence* as well as their previous experience, training and skill. Several studies have found that confidence and competence do not correlate.
- Incompetent subjects overestimate their ability because their incompetence denies them the ability to recognise competence, or lack of it, either in themselves or in others (this is discussed further in Chapter 8).
- There is no evidence that males and females are different in their ability to self-assess, although there is a trend for males to express higher levels of confidence.
- Practical tasks are more amenable to self-assessment than cognitive ones, probably because their outcomes are harder to dispute.
- The factors that improve the ability to self-assess are feedback, increasing knowledge (which increases understanding and recalibration of what good performance involves) and experience.

Some of these concepts are explored in more detail in the next chapter. However, what these themes identify is that self-assessment alone is insufficient as a tool to identify the full extent of one's own learning needs, particularly for trainees. Therefore, trainees need direction as to how to be self-directed.

How can we put a curriculum into practice?

In the light of the above, there are several components to putting a curriculum into practice. These include the following.

- Intentions
  - Clearly understood by all
  - Ensuring that the syllabus is covered
- Processes
  - Trainee and faculty appointments
  - Length and organisation of the programme
  - Trainee and faculty training and support
  - Appraisal
  - Teaching and learning methods
  - Feedback
  - Clinical and educational supervision
  - Mechanisms for dealing with problems
  - Quality control
- Outcomes
  - Trainee assessments
  - Trainee performance

In a programme that is already established, there is also the informal, the hidden and the assessed curricula to consider as they may require corrective action. *Standards* of intentions, outcomes and processes are discussed separately in Chapter 10.

Harden proposed 10 basic questions that should be asked when planning a course or curriculum [15]. They are as follows.

1 What is required as an end product?
2 What are the aims and objectives?
3 What content should be included?
4 How should the content be organised? (e.g. should one topic follow another?)
5 What educational strategies should be adopted?
6 What teaching methods should be used?
7 How should assessment be carried out?
8 How should details of the curriculum be communicated?
9 What educational environment should be fostered?
10 How should the whole process be managed?

The next section describes examples of how some aspects of different curricula in Yorkshire were put into practice: Generic Skills in the Foundation Programme, Flexible Learning for Anaesthetic Trainees (FLAT) and the Yorkshire

Modular Training Programme© in Obstetrics and Gynaecology. They each illustrate how the different components and questions from the above-mentioned lists have been considered and implemented.

Generic skills in the foundation programme

The Leicester, Northampton and Rutland Deanery considered whether or not the foundation programme curriculum could be implemented in 2004 [16]. It asked supervising consultants in a broad range of specialties whether, in their opinion, the foundation 'competencies' could be delivered within the posts available. A number of curriculum domains were identified that could not be delivered within the clinical environment for that specialty. These included 'competencies' in teaching, primary care, mental health and other more focussed parts of the curriculum, including child protection, fitness to drive and some aspects of prescribing.

Dundee Medical School used a questionnaire to survey graduates during their foundation year 1 to enquire what three areas they found most difficult about being a foundation doctor [17]. Although some of the problems highlighted included clinical skills, many of them included elements of the generic content of the curriculum, such as prioritisation, time management, documentation and working with other health professionals.

These two examples illustrate that sometimes the areas in which new doctors need most help in learning are the nonclinical aspects of the curriculum. Formal training days can be a useful means of delivering these more tricky aspects of the curriculum. 'Training days' have subsequently become part of many postgraduate medical education programmes and the content ranges from didactic lectures to more innovative sessions, some of which are described in the following text.

When considering setting up formal training days, it has to be decided whether these can be delivered locally. If the answer is yes, then departments or trusts can be charged with delivering these to their own trainees. However, if the answer is no or if it is uncertain then some additional arrangements may be required to ensure the topics are covered. For example, sections 7 and 8 of the foundation curriculum syllabus are about recognition and management of the acutely ill patient and practical procedures. Most of this is addressed as part of work-based learning; no special arrangements are required. However, the remainder of the syllabus mirrors the General Medical Council's 'Good Medical Practice' [18] and includes generic topics such as time management, patient safety, clinical governance, ethics and legal issues (Box 5.2). In the Yorkshire Deanery, most of these topics required special arrangements because only some teachers were expert in these areas. As a result, throughout the year, trainees attended five training days that covered the generic skills curriculum, each split into half-day sessions delivered by expert teachers.

In the past, most teaching was (and, to some extent, still is) delivered simply by allocating a topic to a speaker and leaving him or her to determine the

Box 5.2 The domains of Good Medical Practice and the foundation
         programme syllabus

- Good clinical care
  - ○ History, examination, diagnosis, record-keeping, safe prescribing
    and reflective practice
  - ○ Time management and decision-making
  - ○ Patient safety
  - ○ Infection control
  - ○ Clinical governance
  - ○ Nutrition care
  - ○ Health promotion, patient education and public health
  - ○ Ethical and legal issues
- Maintaining GMC
  - ○ Learning
  - ○ Research, evidence and guidelines
  - ○ Audit
- Teaching and training
- Relationships with patients and communication skills
- Working with colleagues
- Probity and professional behaviour
- Personal health

Appraising and assessing is included in Good Medical Practice but not
the foundation programme syllabus.

content and teaching methods to be used. However, teaching and *learning*
are not the same thing. It is important to design formal training days with
educational principles in mind, if they are to be of any value to learners.

Teaching methods are beyond the scope of this chapter. However, one
example of a different way of organising a training day is the SCORPIO system of medical teaching [19]. Developed for undergraduate medical education, this system addresses many of the criticisms of traditional medical
education and stands for: Structured, Clinical, Objective Referenced, Problem-
based, Integrated and Organised. It involves delivering a particular part of a
syllabus in a setting similar to a training day. At the start, a short lecture gives
an overview of the topic and then students or trainees rotate around a series
of teaching stations in small groups. The learning objectives for each station
are clearly displayed. A wide range of resource material can be used, including patients (or simulated patients), medical equipment, test results and scenarios for discussion. Each station is staffed by the most appropriate teacher.
Assessment can be built into the day if needed. While they may not be
labelled with this particular acronym, several training days in our region have
been designed using this model, including 'critical care for surgical SHOs',

'acute care training (ACT)' for foundation year 1 doctors, and training days in the Yorkshire Modular Training Programme©.

Flexible Learning for Anaesthetic Trainees (FLAT)

In common with most specialist training programmes, the Pennine School of Anaesthesia ran formal training days that were compulsory for trainees preparing for their final FRCA examination. These training days consisted of didactic lectures, a form of teaching that is least effective in terms of learning, and mock examinations at the end of each year. With the introduction of the European Working Time Directive, attendance at this type of programme became a problem and the course was reviewed.

The new course was designed with Harden's 10 basic questions in mind. It had to be flexible and the quality had to be high, yet the organisers wanted to retain the sense of community that existed among trainees working towards their final FRCA examination [20].

In this case, the end product, objectives and content were clear. Content was divided into five blocks (e.g. Block 1 – intensive care, resuscitation and trauma). The course was developed by a small team of people with qualifications and expertise in medical education and e-learning. Didactic lectures were replaced with 'blended learning' – a mixture of Web-based material (interactive lectures, patient management problems, online discussion board, reading material and links to relevant external learning sources) and less frequent blocks of face-to-face teaching that consisted of interactive group tutorials. In some cases, homework was provided on the Web beforehand and trainees were asked to prepare material for discussion during these sessions, which were designed to expand on the Web-based learning and further explore difficult concepts, rather than simply repeat topics. The process was managed by the local academic unit of anaesthesia, helped by funding from the Yorkshire Deanery.

E-learning has become popular in recent years because of the limitations of the European Working Time Directive, the introduction of competency-based training, the accessibility of the Internet and the ability to reach large numbers of learners 'any time, any place' [21]. It is discussed further in Chapter 9. Much of what trainees in medicine learn is encountered during clinical practice. The downside of this is that 'such knowledge may remain tacit or disconnected from other knowledge, or difficult to apply in future. To be most fruitful, opportunistic learning must be integrated with other experiences and then generalised so that it is not tied to a single context or incident' [22]. If educationally well designed and integrated into a curriculum that includes other forms of learning, e-learning can be a valuable tool (see Chapter 9).

The Yorkshire Modular Training Programme

The limitations of the European Working Time Directive and the introduction of competency-based training were also some of the drivers for a 'modular' approach to implementing the specialist training curriculum in obstetrics and gynaecology.

A module in this context is a 'short unit, complete in itself, which may be linked to further units towards the achievement of larger tasks or long-term goals'. The curriculum was organised into five major modules, to be covered in each year of training [23]. The advantages and disadvantages of such a system were described by the organisers and are shown in Box 5.3.

Box 5.3

Advantages and disadvantages of a modular approach to putting a curriculum into practice.

Advantages	Disadvantages
A coherent continuum for trainees, avoiding repetition or gaps	A problem if trainees move in or out of the region
Clear aims and objectives for each module – for trainers and trainees	Some trainees need support in taking greater responsibility for their own learning
Allows trainers to teach to their strengths	
Teaching material and organisation produced only once and then updated from time to time	
All obstetrics and gynaecology units in the region participate	

This particular modular programme used the SPICES model to address curriculum development [24] and encouraged a student-centred, problem- and community-orientated, systematic approach – see Box 5.4. Within each module, a range of formal teaching activities were organised, including homework,

---

Box 5.4 The SPICES model

This model lists six issues that curriculum planners need to take into account. Each issue is presented as a spectrum between two extremes. On the left are the more innovative approaches (SPICES), and on the

(*Continued*)

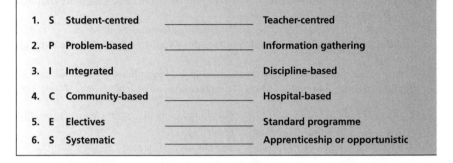

Box 5.4 (Continued)

right are the more traditional strategies. Decisions about where on the continuum a particular curriculum should sit will depend on a number of factors.

1.	S	Student-centred	_____ Teacher-centred
2.	P	Problem-based	_____ Information gathering
3.	I	Integrated	_____ Discipline-based
4.	C	Community-based	_____ Hospital-based
5.	E	Electives	_____ Standard programme
6.	S	Systematic	_____ Apprenticeship or opportunistic

small group work, skills training, courses, e-learning and conferences. The overall programme was supported by a well-organised administrative structure that included 'tracking' of individual trainees through the programme.

Overall, this modular approach led to more structured processes in the curriculum, including quality control. Teaching across a region became standardised. However, the organisers of this programme themselves admit that postgraduate medical trainees have been used to more traditional and passive methods of teaching, such as lectures, and some have needed support while engaging in more active forms of learning.

Conclusions

Putting a curriculum into practice in postgraduate medical education presents us with a much greater challenge than previously. In many specialties there was no formal curriculum. The knowledge, skills and attitudes that trainees are required to attain today include not only clinical topics but also generic ones – subject areas that are as important but sometimes outside natural areas of expertise of the clinicians. However, by understanding that a curriculum includes *everything* that happens in relation to an educational programme, and how it happens, putting a curriculum into practice allows for more creativity on our part in its development and delivery.

References

1. Postgraduate Medical Education and Training Board. What is a curriculum? URL www.pmetb.org.uk/fileadmin/user/Communications/Publications/PMETB_what_is_curriculum.pdf

2. Fish D, Coles C. Medical education, developing a curriculum for practice. Open University Press, Maidenhead, 2005.
3. Talbot M. Monkey see, monkey do. A critique of the competency model in graduate medical education. *Med Educ* 2004; **38**: 587–592.
4. Talbot M. Good wine may need to mature: a critique of accelerated higher specialist training. Evidence from cognitive neuroscience. *Med Educ* 2004; **38**: 399–408.
5. ten Cate O. Trust, competence, and the supervisor's role in postgraduate training. *BMJ* 2006; **333**: 748–751.
6. Ericsson KA. Deliberate practice and the acquisition and maintenance of expert performance in medicine and related domains. *Acad Med* 2004; **79 (10 Suppl.)**: S70–S81.
7. Lempp H, Seale C. The hidden curriculum in undergraduate medical education: qualitative study of medical students' perceptions of teaching. *BMJ* 2004; **329**: 770–773.
8. Davies M. Principles of curriculum development. University of Dundee Masters Programme in Medical Education, Dundee, 2003.
9. Academy of Medical Royal Colleges and the Departments of Health. Foundation Programme curriculum. AoMRC, London, 2007. URL www.foundationprogramme.nhs.uk
10. Harth SC, Bavanandan S, Thomas KE, Lai MY, Thong YH. The quality of student–tutor interactions in the clinical learning environment. *Med Educ* 1992; **26**: 321–326.
11. Robbins LS, Gruppen LD, Alexander GL, Fantone JC, Davis WK. A predictive model of student satisfaction with the medical school learning environment. *Acad Med* 1997; **72 (2)**: 134–139.
12. Herzberg F. Work and the nature of man. New American Library, New York, 1966.
13. Postgraduate Medical Education Training Board/General Medical Council. Standards for training for the Foundation Training Programme, 2007. URL www.pmetb.org.uk/fileadmin/user/QA/QAFP/Standards_for_Training_270307.pdf
14. Colthart I, Bagnall G, Evans A, *et al*. The effectiveness of self-assessment on the identification of learner needs, learner activity, and impact on clinical practice: BEME (Best Evidence Medical Education) Guide no. 10. *Med Teach* 2008; **30**: 124–145.
15. Harden RM. Ten questions to ask when planning a course or curriculum. *Med Educ* 1986; **20**: 356–365.
16. Higgins R, Cavendish S. Modernising Medical Careers. Foundation Programme curriculum competencies: will all rotations allow the necessary skills to be acquired? The consultants' predictions. *Postgrad Med J* 2006; **82**: 684–687.
17. McIlwaine L, Jarvis RI, Kerr JS. What do recently qualified doctors think would help prepare medical students for Foundation Year 1? In: Monograph on the Foundation Programme. ASME, Edinburgh, 2007.
18. General Medical Council. Good Medical Practice. GMC, London, 2006. URL www.gmc-uk.org
19. Hill DA. SCORPIO – a system of medical teaching. *Med Teach* 1992; **14 (1)**: 37–41.
20. Forrest K, Smith S, Howell S. A new way of learning – reflections on our first year. Bulletin 28. The Royal College of Anaesthetists, November 2004. URL www.rcoa.ac.uk/docs/Bulletin28.pdf
21. McKendree J. Understanding medical education. E learning. Association for the Study of Medical Education, Edinburgh, 2006.

22. Davies M, Forrest K. E learning. In: How to teach continuing medical education. Wiley-Blackwell, Oxford, 2008.
23. Duffy S, Jha V, Kaufmann S. The Yorkshire Modular Training Programme: a model for structured training and quality assurance in obstetrics and gynaecology. *Med Teach* 2004; **26 (6)**: 540–544.
24. Harden RM, Sowden S, Dunn WR. Some educational strategies in curriculum development: the SPICES model. Association for the Study of Medical Education booklet no. 18. ASME, Edinburgh, 1984.
25. Cooper (2007), with permission from Association for the Study of Medical Education (ASME). The Foundation Programme curriculum – where to now? In: Monograph on the Foundation Programme. ASME, Edinburgh, 2007.

Further resources

- Postgraduate Medical Education Training Board. Standards for curricula. PMETB, London, 2005. URL www.pmetb.org.uk/fileadmin/user/Communications/Publications/PMETB_standards_for_curricula__March_2005_.pdf
- Postgraduate Medical Education Training Board. Standards for curriculum development: background paper. PMETB, London, 2005. URL www.pmetb.org.uk/fileadmin/user/Communications/Publications/PMETB_background_paper_-_standards_for_curriculum_development__September_2004_.pdf

CHAPTER 6
Teaching and learning

Kirsty Forrest[1] & Sean Williamson[2]
[1]The Leeds Teaching Hospitals NHS Trust, Leeds, UK
[2]The James Cook University Hospital, Middlesborough, UK

'How can we teach our students if we do not know how they learn?' [1]

The interest in this question is not merely medical but encompasses all of education. Much of the research on learning relates to university education, although there is considerable interest from medical educators and business leaders as well. The previous chapter dealt with the 'big picture' of an educational programme. This chapter focuses on teaching and learning at a more individual level, starting with the nature of professional education, the use of opportunistic teaching methods and then some common models of adult learning and how these can be applied to postgraduate medical education.

Professional education

Learning is 'internalisation of knowledge' and professional education is a mixture of learning from:
- daily work (e.g. ward rounds, theatre, outpatients);
- debriefing and reflection;
- written or web-based material;
- formal teaching sessions (e.g. meetings, lectures and courses);
- projects.

The foundation programme curriculum, for example, emphasises that doctors learn in and from the practice of medicine [2]. Teaching is guiding this learning and aiding the acquisition of knowledge, skills, attitudes and behaviours.

Shorter, more focussed, competency-based training in postgraduate medical education is not without controversy. Doctors are required to pursue an extensive period of training following initial qualification, which involves scholarly understanding as well as technical training, work-based learning, postgraduate courses and examinations. However, the practice of medicine

Essential Guide to Educational Supervision in Postgraduate Medical Education.
Edited by Nicola Cooper and Kirsty Forrest. © 2009 Blackwell Publishing,
ISBN: 978-1-4051-7071-0.

is much more than a set of predetermined tasks carried out by highly trained technicians.

'Competent' is a legal term that refers to being adequately qualified [3]. In everyday use this is understood to mean 'good enough', but as Sir John Tooke wrote in his foreword to the Independent Inquiry into Modernising Medical Careers (MMC), 'In reflecting on the evidence it received and formulating its recommendations, the Independent Inquiry Panel was clear: mechanisms that smacked of an aspiration to mediocrity were inadmissible. Put simply, 'good enough' is not good enough. Rather, in the interests of the health and wealth of the nation, we should aspire to excellence' [4].

How do we aim for excellence as the goal of postgraduate medical education? There is a wealth of literature on this subject and this chapter will recap some of the main points.

There are some key factors that help people develop expert professional practice (excellence). These are:
- experience;
- feedback;
- deliberate practice;
- reflection.

These are all areas that educational supervisors and training programme directors can make explicit, facilitate and coach trainees in.

Experience

For most everyday activities, such as driving a car or playing tennis, an acceptable standard of performance is usually attained within less than 50h of practice. For professional practice, the time frame is in years. Research in sports, sciences and arts shows that performers need a minimum of 10 years of intense involvement before they can reach an expert level [5].

This has implications for postgraduate medical education. Although it may vary from person to person, it appears that there is a minimum amount of time, or number of cases to be seen, required to reach an expert level of performance.

Feedback

However, hours worked and the number of cases seen are not enough. Consistent gradual improvement in performance also requires feedback. It is possible to have lots of experience in doing something the wrong way. Without an expert to give feedback on your performance you cannot improve, as you 'don't know what you don't know'. Feedback in itself has been subject to much research. For feedback to be educationally effective, it has to be:
- interactive (including a self-assessment and development of an action plan by the learner);
- based on direct observation;
- constructive;
- close in time to the observed event;

- specific;
- consistent (not conflicting with previous information);
- face to face;
- receivable [6].

The sources of this feedback can be varied – it is not always that the most senior clinician provides the best feedback. In the absence of external feedback, sometimes it is, 'What you get when you don't get what you expected'.

Surveys of trainees consistently show that feedback, as perceived by them, is not a common experience. In one study, 80% of the trainees reported never or infrequently receiving corrective feedback from their consultants, 20% reported sometimes receiving corrective feedback, and none reported receiving it often [7]. Yet adult learners in theory welcome feedback, especially when it is based on their performance and tailored to their goals. Educational research suggests that teachers should create an appropriate learning environment (discussed in the previous chapter), orientate trainees to the focus of the session, elicit their knowledge, skills and attitudes during the session, give appropriate feedback and then summarise the session at the end to check understanding [8]. How this very simple educational model can be incorporated into work-based learning is described later.

Deliberate practice

Experience and feedback are good, but not good enough if we aspire to excellence. Deliberate practice is also required. This refers to time spent on a specific activity designed to improve performance in a particular aspect of practice. Several studies have found a consistent association between the amount and the quality of deliberate practice and performance in domains as varied as chess, music and sport. Deliberate practice means that there is effort involved as well as some form of feedback, whether through self-assessment or observation by another person.

The relationship between deliberate practice and performance has been studied in medicine. One study describes how accuracy of diagnosis is related to the training and the experience of the subjects – but in two different ways (see Figure 6.1) [5]. Recordings of heart sounds were played to physicians and medical students. Experience and continuing training (specialisation) correlated with improved performance, but experience without continuing training resulted in a gradual decrease in performance. In other words, continuing training is important for performance. This has also been shown in other areas such as dermatology, electrocardiogram interpretation and histopathology. Short-term training courses are not the same as deliberate practice and do not have the same beneficial effects on long-term performance.

Research on laparoscopic trainers and other simulators shows that structured practice with feedback on a simulator improves subsequent performance in the same real-life situation (e.g. knot-tying skills). Deliberate practice using simulation is particularly useful for new skills, rare events or emergencies.

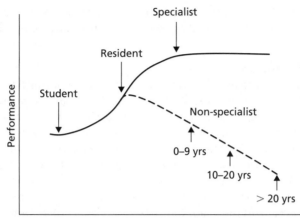

Figure 6.1 Performance in relation to continuing training and experience. Reproduced with permission from Ericsson KA. Deliberate practice and the acquisition and maintenance of expert performance in medicine and related domains. *Academic Medicine* 2004; 79(10): S70–S81 [5].

Reflection

Reflection is a vital aspect of developing expert professional practice. Chapter 7 describes reflection-in-action (thinking on our feet) and reflection-on-action (thinking, talking or writing afterwards) described by Schön, and then goes on to discuss narrative reflection, which is one form of reflection.

Some people are naturally reflective, but everyone can be helped to reflect in a more practical and structured way. Reflective practice is when we view our practice from different perspectives: our own experiences, our colleagues' or patients' experiences and perceptions, and the literature. In some ways, this process is a bit like the audit cycle. Of course, it applies to educational supervisors as well.

Reflection is how we 'cook' raw feedback and direct experience into an integrated, internalised source of clinical judgement and skills.

How to 'teach' excellence

Educational supervisors should be able to explain the concepts outlined in the preceding text to their trainees, and help them engage in activities that will develop their own expert professional practice – or identify someone else who can. A key role of the educational supervisor is in guiding learning and there are many courses, societies and publications available to support this (see further resources).

Most of postgraduate medical education is delivered in the workplace. In 2002, the Conference of Postgraduate Medical Deans (COPMeD) published *Liberating Learning*, intended as a practical guide for teaching and learning in the context of the European Working Time Directive. The guide lists over 30 different activities that can be used as part of work-based learning [9].

Opportunistic teaching

Guiding learning as part of daily work is known as opportunistic teaching, and several different models exist. As Osler said, 'There should be no teaching without the patient for a text and the best teaching is often that taught by the patient himself' [10]. Some of these models overlap with the work-based assessments that are now in common use in postgraduate medical education. As an educational supervisor, being aware of these models can help you in your role as a teacher.

A common misconception is that opportunistic teaching requires no planning. However, without planning there is a danger that clinicians will teach their favourite subjects repeatedly to the same trainees. Preparation includes:
- knowing the curriculum;
- knowing the learners (so that teaching is targeted);
- setting mutual goals.

Another common misperception is that there is not enough time to teach when the focus is meant to be on patient care. Some clinicians find that teaching on a ward round or in clinic, for example, takes too much time and therefore feel they can only focus on patient care or teaching, but not both at the same time. This is where understanding some of the models described later can help.

These methods of opportunistic teaching are underpinned by educational principles and are designed to be incorporated into daily work. It is not an exhaustive list, but a common theme is that many of these models are about making the implicit knowledge of the teacher more explicit to the trainee.

Demonstrations by the teacher

Demonstrations are what many clinicians do all the time in their clinical practice. However, without making it clear to the trainee that this is a training episode, a learning opportunity can be missed. This can be as simple as stating something like, 'I would like you to watch how I take a history/ examine the patient/perform this procedure. Concentrate on what questions I ask/what I look for/how I interact with theatre colleagues. Afterwards I would like you to summarise what you observed and then we will discuss it further'.

In this method of opportunistic teaching, the teacher has to be open to honest feedback from the trainee, and not get too dispirited when what seems obvious is not quite grasped by the trainee – this can be a particular problem when the learning is focussed on less tangible subjects such as clinical reasoning or team working. These subjects may be better taught by the next method.

The expert 'thinking aloud'

As experts, some of our clinical judgements can appear to be so intuitive as to be unteachable. As a teacher you may be asked how you just 'knew' something. This is a bit like trying to explain how you drive a car, broken down into its constituent parts, and can be difficult. In the previous system of postgraduate medical education, trainees learned from multiple examples over more years and more hours worked per week. Shorter, more structured training programmes mean that teachers need to facilitate learning in a more focussed way. One way is by making explicit the steps that you have gone through to get to a particular endpoint.

Sound clinical reasoning and judgement at critical points in time is a valuable skill for trainees to learn. How did you know that the patient was sick? The answer of 'gut feeling' is not helpful to trainees and is not supported by the literature on expert practice. Gut feelings usually involve the immediate recognition of a constellation of signs (visual, auditory etc.) that fit into a pattern that matches with your previous experience.

Often, as a clinical teacher, the simple act of thinking aloud can help trainees to understand the steps you are taking when coming to a decision and management plan, and this facilitates learning.

Observation with feedback

Structured observation of trainees should involve some planning, with an explanation to all involved including the patient. Work-based assessments are discussed further in Chapter 9, including the importance of assessor training. These assessments are designed to be trainee-led, with the trainee initiating the experience of being observed and assessed. However, this does not stop teachers from taking the initiative as well. For example, 'This ward round/clinic is an opportunity for us to do a mini-CEX if you would like'.

Work-based assessments are designed for two purposes: to identify doctors in difficulty and (more commonly) to provide opportunities for feedback on the performance of trainees so that they can improve their practice.

Teaching in chunks

Many models of 'quick' teaching are documented in the literature [11]. These include the 'One Minute Preceptor Model', which is a way of incorporating teaching into a patient-focussed clinical encounter. It involves trainees presenting a case they have seen and then:
- getting an idea about what the trainees think is going on with the patient;
- probing their reasoning and alternative explanations;
- teaching one or two general principles;
- giving positive feedback about what the trainee did well;
- correcting any errors in reasoning.

Other methods of teaching in 'quick digestible chunks' include asking questions, reviewing patients that the trainee has seen and then discussing your diagnosis and management plan, and the SNAPPS model (developed for outpatient clinics – summarise, narrow down, analyse the differentials, probe the teacher about uncertainties, plan the patient's management and then select a topic for self-directed learning related to the case).

These teaching methods provide a way of teaching when the focus is on patient care. Small chunks of teaching can be very effective, particularly when they are set in an overall context in which trainees are expected to participate in learning. Remember, teaching and learning are not the same thing. Box 6.1 summarises the steps to consider when planning patient-centred teaching [12].

Box 6.1 Key steps to consider when planning patient-centred teaching (Reprinted with permission from [12])

Before

        Preparation
        Planning
        Orientation

During

        Introduction
        Interaction
        Observation
        Instruction
        Summarising

After

        Debriefing
        Feedback
        Reflection
        Preparation

Role modelling

Role modelling is teaching by example. Poor role modelling can have a powerful impact on the informal and hidden curricula, which are described in Chapter 5. There are three categories of role modelling in medicine [13].
- Clinical competence
- Teaching skills
- Personal qualities (e.g. compassion, integrity, enthusiasm, quest for excellence)

Role modelling is a good way to demonstrate professional behaviour and can be used to teach other aspects of patient care, for example infection prevention and communication skills. Many doctors in difficulty may be perpetuating behaviour they have observed go unchallenged in senior colleagues.

The humanistic side of medicine is something that is valued by patients and trainees alike.

Assessing competence and excellence

Another approach towards how to 'teach' excellence is emphasising that there are many ways to teach and assess trainees. Hodges describes how we think of medical education as a process that moves trainees from a state of incompetence to competence. However, competence can be conceptualised in different ways, and if we emphasise one form of teaching and assessing over another we can actually create incompetence as a side-effect [14].

After analysing the medical education literature on competence, four main discourses were identified.
- Competence as knowledge
- Competence as performance
- Competence as a reliable test score
- Competence as a reflective practitioner

If trainees are taught and assessed in only one of these discourses, there is a danger of creating a one-dimensional doctor. Box 6.2 shows the four discourses and the hidden problems that can arise if competence is emphasised in this area alone. Assessment methods are usually decided by policymakers, but teachers can vary the ways in which they impart knowledge, skills and attitudes and assess these parameters in their own trainees.

From teacher- to learner-centred

There are two different foci in any teaching encounter. The teacher may become the centre of the group and assume formal authority and control the information delivered. This is very much the style of a lecturer. Another teacher-centred style involves demonstration and personal delivery of what is expected from the learner. This is very much the style of apprenticeship, which involves acting as a role model and coach to the learner.

However, in shifting the focus to the learner our teaching style needs to facilitate and focus activities. Learners need initiative and independence to function effectively in this learning environment either in a group or as an individual. They also need to develop together. Although this is a style more suited to adult learning, it is variable in junior doctors as to how far they can all learn this way. The effectiveness of a group in this situation is dependent on the interpersonal relationship of the group.

Work-based learning relies on both the apprenticeship style as well as the learner-centred one in which the learner invites the teacher to guide training encounters. However, there are different stages of knowledge and skill acquisition, described by Dreyfuss (see Box 6.3); therefore, the teacher needs to know at what stage the trainee is and teach accordingly [15].

Box 6.2

Discourses in competence (Reprinted with permission from [14])

Discourse	Role of teacher	Role of student	Measure	Hidden problems
Knowledge	Knowledge giver	Memorising and recall	Multiple choice and other examinations	Inability to recognise patterns Poor technical and interpersonal skills
Performance	Skills teacher	Practicing and demonstrating skills	Simulation, objective structured clinical examinations	Lack of integration of knowledge with performance. 'Fake' performances
Reliable test score	Preparing students for standard assessments	Maximising scores on standardised measures	Standardised tests (e.g. objective structured clinical examinations)	Prolongation of novice behaviours (e.g. scattergun approach to history taking) and inability to deal with variation Lack of development of expert reasoning skills
Reflective practitioner	Guiding introspection, mentor	Self-assessment and self-direction	Portfolios	Superficial self-assessment Development of reflective ability alone in the absence of knowledge and skills

Box 6.3

Skill acquisition (Dreyfuss)

Level 1	Novice	Little or no experience, goal oriented, lacking judgement, rigid adherence to rules or plans
Level 2	Advanced beginner	Starts tasks alone but cannot solve variation. Looks for rapid reward. Can follow guidelines without necessarily understanding. All attributes given equal importance
Level 3	Competent	Has conceptual models, identifies problems, seeks expert advice
Level 4	Proficient	Sees situations holistically, applies previous experience and the experiences of others. Can rationalise even small details
Level 5	Expert	No longer needs guidelines, works off intuition and only applies principles to solve new variations. Following rules reduces performance

The next section describes the principles of adult learning and some commonly described learning styles, and how these theories can be applied to postgraduate medical education.

Principles of adult learning

The term 'andragogy' (meaning the art and science of helping adults learn) was coined in the 1980s and is based on a set of assumptions that centre around the fact that adults tend to be independent and self-directed learners. The characteristics of adult learning are listed as follows.
- They are self-directed rather than dependent, and are capable of determining their own learning needs and of finding the means to meet them.
- They have accumulated experience, which is a resource for learning and can provide a context for that learning.
- They value learning that is closely related to their own personal development or goals.
- They value knowledge that can be applied, rather than learning for the sake of learning.
- They tend to be motivated by internal factors (e.g. desire to succeed) more than external ones.

With this in mind, teachers need to recognise that adults tend to disengage or perform poorly during learning activities that ignore their previous experience and personal goals or are not demonstrably applicable to their everyday work. Therefore, involving learners in planning learning objectives, methods and evaluation may result in a more successful teaching programme.

Learning styles

Undoubtedly there are different ways of learning. One theory is that under-standing different learning styles may help to develop more effective teaching strategies.

Any group will contain a complete spectrum of learning style preferences. The ideal teacher should be able to adapt to all styles. Failure to align course delivery to different methods of learning may simply lead to wastage of time. Therefore, course design should seek to reinforce each key point in three or four different ways. A good example of this is the current adult life support courses. The concept that delivering early defibrillation is essential is taught in pre-course reading for the visual learner, in a lecture for the auditory learner and in workshops for the hands-on learner. All of this is on a background of motivation that failure to comply with the course material may lead to failure in career progression. The literature on this topic is varied and extensive.

Families of learning styles

Several different terminologies are in use when it comes to learning styles, and the science is derived from the social sciences and psychology, which may be unfamiliar to doctors. Notable and useful examples exist within each family of learning styles.

Mind styles

Hermann proposed that there is left or right brain dominance [16]. The right-brained learner likes pictures, charts, activities and music whereas the left-brained learner prefers reading, writing, details and organisation. The implications for teaching are straightforward, that both styles should be catered for.

Another simple way of thinking about mind styles is by using the acronym VARK. This stands for:
- visual (diagrams and images);
- auditory (listening and discussion);
- reading (and writing in all its forms);
- kinaesthetic (sensory or hands-on).

Again, using a range of teaching methods in an educational programme is likely to be more effective in facilitating learning across a group.

Personality type

Thousands of articles have been written on the Myers–Briggs Type Indicator MBTI® [17], which focuses on the fact that personality type influences the way people prefer to absorb information, make decisions and communicate.

Box 6.4 The four dimensions of the MBTI

1. How a person energises
   Extraversion (in the outer world) ↔ Introversion (in the inner world)
2. How a person takes in information
   Sensing (through their senses, doers) ↔ Intuition (through seeing the big picture, imaginers)
3. How a person makes decisions
   Thinking (fact analysis, task orientated) ↔ Feeling (values analysis, people orientated)
4. How a person organises himself
   Judging (organised, enjoy completing) ↔ Perceiving (flexible, enjoy the process)

Thus, there are 16 different possible MBTI personality types, all subtly different.

In the MBTI, four basic dimensions of personality are described (see Box 6.4). This indicator is increasingly used by institutions to assess, strengths and weaknesses in the context of teams.

Experiential learning

One of the most influential models of learning was developed by Kolb in the early 1970s. His theory of experiential learning and the instrument that he devised to test it have generated a considerable body of research, which suggests that learning is best achieved in an environment that considers both concrete experiences and conceptual models [18]. Kolb's four learning environments are:

- abstract conceptualisation – learning by thinking;
- active experimentation – learning by doing;
- concrete experience – learning by feeling;
- reflective observation – learning by reflection, watching and listening.

Honey and Mumford [19] built on Kolb's idea that people tend to prefer different methods of learning, but rather than seeing people as at opposite ends of a spectrum, they believed that people move between these four different states of learning, which they termed activist, reflector, theorist and pragmatist. In their model, learners have an experience, reflect on it, draw their own conclusions (theorise) and then put the theory into practice to see what happens.

These concepts are illustrated further in Figure 6.2 and Box 6.5.

Many of the learning styles can be assessed using questionnaires that are available to help individuals discern their own learning preferences. Learning styles are only models designed to help, not pigeonhole, the learning process. For teachers, the relevance of understanding learning styles is that we tend to plan and teach in our own style. In theory, we can vary the style within a programme to engage more learners and maximise learning.

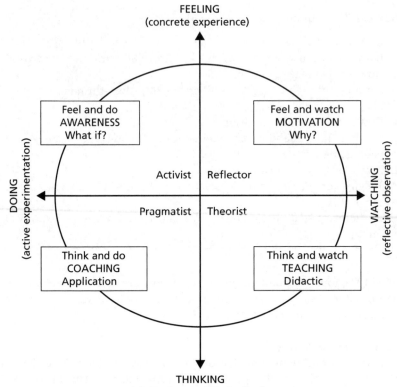

Figure 6.2 The learning cycle and learning styles.
Reproduced with permission by Blackwell Publishing from Cooper N, Forrest K and Cramp P. Learning about learning. In: Essential Guide to Generic Skills. Blackwell Publishing, Oxford, 2006.

In Figure 6.2, the cycle represents the process of learning. For example, imagine you are give the task of teaching a small group of doctors how to perform a lumbar puncture. The cycle helps to explain the process that learners need to go through in order to learn successfully. This process need not start at any point but includes theory, coaching (which could include simulation), 'real life' activity and reflection.

At every stage, there will be people who prefer to learn in a certain way. Some will prefer theory whereas other will prefer practice. The reality is they need all stages to learn effectively. This model can be applied to almost any subject, not just practical procedures.

Learning strategies
A related concept is that learners can choose to learn different things in different ways depending on the nature of their need and motivations. Merely liking the course or being driven by an impending examination can drive

Box 6.5

How different learning styles like to learn and teach

Learning style	Characteristic strengths of each learning style	Activities that support that learning style	Activities as a teacher with that learning style
People who like to feel and watch (reflectors)	Imaginative ability and generation of ideas	Investigations and puzzles Reading and essay writing Use of the library, factual research Lectures Tests	Acts as a transmitter to further students within the discipline
People who like to think and watch (theorists)	Creating theoretical models and making sense of disparate observations	Problem solving Role-playing Making and constructing Writing for an audience Wide variety of media, for example video, internet, music	Acts as a manager to prepare students to perform the skills in the real world
People who like to think and do (pragmatists)	Practical application of ideas	Group work Broad brief with choices Presentations Opportunity to make mistakes	Acts as a colleague to enhance the student's vision of what could be achievable
People who like to feel and do (activists)	Carrying out plans and tasks that involve them in new experiences	Debate Conversations Structured group work Peer teaching and learning Opportunities to hypothesise, ask questions and use imagination	Acts as a facilitator to further student growth and development

Reproduced with permission by Blackwell/Publishing from Ref. [20].

learners to undertake an unwitting cost–benefit analysis of the best way to approach the topics at hand.

Strategies may be divided into two distinct groups.

- Serialists follow a step-by-step sequence, concentrating on narrow hypotheses taking one step at a time. Learning is very contextual and problems may be met by failing to understand the whole picture.
- Holists form complex hypotheses relating to more than one idea and seek patterns and analogies to give explanation and structure to learning. Thus, learning is by understanding. The opposite problems may exist, in that overgeneralisation and loss of detail is possible.

Other learning strategies involve deep or surface learning. Deep learning involves the critical analysis of new ideas, linking them to already known concepts and principles, and leads to understanding and long-term retention of concepts so that they can be used for problem solving in unfamiliar contexts. Deep learning promotes understanding and application. By contrast, surface learning is the tacit acceptance of information and memorisation as isolated and unlinked facts. It leads to superficial retention of material and does not promote understanding or long-term retention of knowledge. This is a common approach to examination preparation with lists of differential diagnoses and is characteristic of the novice.

Although the teacher's perception of surface learning is bad, it is the learner's perception that passing knowledge-based assessments is good. Influencing these learning approaches is key to successful teaching in professional education where deep learning is important (see Box 6.6). Major influences on approaches to learning are assessment methods. Short questions testing separate ideas encourage surface learning. The foundation curriculum design and assessment tools, for example, are meant to encourage a deeper approach.

Box 6.6

Deep learning versus surface learning

	Deep learning	Surface learning
Definition	Examining new facts and ideas critically, tying them into existing cognitive structures and making numerous links between ideas	Accepting new facts and ideas uncritically and attempting to store them as isolated, unconnected, items
Characteristics	Looks for meaning and concepts connecting different topics using evidence and previous knowledge to link learning to real life	Uses rote learning and rigid formulae, failing to give weight to information or incorporate previous work in order to learn for an examination

(Continued)

Box 6.6 (Continued)

Student features	Curious, knowledgeable, confident, good time management, likes education environment	Examination motivation, lacking understanding, numerous time conflicts with work or home, believing that factual recall is what is required
Teacher features	Interested, versatile, in-depth knowledge, consistent. Uses key concepts, relates material and relates assessments. Mistakes allowed. Uses structure	Uninterested, negative, hurried. Poor structure with information overload. Focus on frequent testing

Conclusions

The word 'doctor' comes from the Latin *docere* meaning 'to teach'. All doctors are teachers, but not all doctors know how to teach or guide learning.

Chapter 5 discusses the role of the trainee in learning, including the limitations of trainees to be truly self-directed. In this chapter, we have discussed how educational supervisors can guide learning, by understanding, making explicit and, in some cases, modelling what we have described in the preceding text.

References

1. Dunn R, Dunn K. Teaching secondary students through their individual learning styles. Needham Heights, Allyn and Bacon, 1992.
2. Academy of Medical Royal Colleges and the Departments of Health. Foundation Programme Curriculum, 2007. www.foundationprogramme.nhs.uk
3. Armitage M, Raza TH. Modernising Medical Careers: the need to isolate myths from facts. *Clin Teacher* 2008; **5**: 19–22.
4. Tooke J, Ashtiany S, Carter D *et al*. Aspiring to excellence. Findings and final recommendations of the independent inquiry into Modernising Medical Careers. MMC Inquiry, London, 2008. www.mmcinquiry.org.uk
5. Ericsson KA. Deliberate practice and the acquisition and maintenance of expert performance in medicine and related domains. *Acad Med* 2004; **79 (10)**: S70–S81.
6. Cooper N, Forrest K, Cramp P (Eds). How to give feedback. In: Essential guide to generic skills. Blackwell/BMJ, Oxford, 2006.
7. Isaacson JH, Posk LK, Litaker DG, Halperin AK. Resident perceptions of the evaluation process. *J Gen Intern Med* 1995; **10 (Suppl.)**: 89.
8. Hewson MG, Little ML. Giving feedback in medical education. Verification of recommended techniques. *J Gen Intern Med* 1998; **13 (2)**: 111–116.
9. Report of COPMeD's ad hoc working group on the educational implications of the European Working Time Directive. Liberating Learning – a practical guide for learners and teachers to postgraduate medical education and the European Working Time Directive. COPMeD, London, 2002. www.copmed.org.uk

10. Bliss M. William Osler: a life in medicine. Oxford University Press, New York, 1999.
11. Irby DM, Wilkerson L. Teaching when time is limited. *Br Med J* 2008; **336**: 384–387.
12. Ramani S. Twelve tips to improve bedside teaching. *Med Teacher* 2003; **25 (2)**: 112.
13. Cruess SR, Cruess RL, Steinert Y. Role modelling. *Br Med J* 2008; **336**: 718–721.
14. Hodges, B. Medical education and the maintenance of incompetence. *Med Teacher* 2006; **28 (8)**: 690.
15. Dreyfuss H, Dreyfuss S. Mind over machine: the power of human intuition and expertise in the era of the computer. Basil Blackwell, Oxford, 1986.
16. Hermann N. The creative brain books. The Ned Hermann Group, Lake Lure, NC, 1989.
17. Myers I, McCauley M. Manual: a guide to the development and use of Myers–Briggs type indicator. Palo Alto Consulting Psychologists Press, Palo Alto, CA, 1985.
18. Kolb D. Facilitator's guide to learning. Hat/McBer, Boston, 2000.
19. Honey P, Mumford A. The manual of learning styles. Peter Honey Publications Ltd, Maidenhead, 1992.
20. Cooper N, Forrest K and Cramp P. Learning about learning. In: Essential guide to generic skills. Blackwell/Publishing, Oxford, 2006.

Further resources

- Newble D, Cannon R. A handbook for medical teachers, 4th edition. Kluwer Academic Publishers, Dordrecht, the Netherlands, 2001.
- Fish D, De Cossart L. Developing the wise doctor: a resource for trainers and trainees (in practice). Royal Society of Medicine Press Ltd, London, 2007.
- De Cossart L, Fish D. Cultivating a thinking surgeon: new perspectives on clinical teaching, learning and assessment. TFM Publishing Ltd, London, 2005.
- Ramani S, Leinster S. AMEE Guide no 34: teaching in the clinical environment. *Med Teacher* 2008; **30**: 347–364.
- Davis M, Forrest K. How to teach continuing medical education. Wiley-Blackwell, 2008.
- Kaufman DM, Mann KV. Teaching and learning in medical education: how theory can inform practice. Association of Medical Education [understanding medical education series], London, 2007. www.asme.org.uk

Organisations

- Association for the Study of Medical Education (ASME). www.asme.org.uk
- Association for Medical Education in Europe (AMEE). www.amee.org
- Academy of Medical Educators. A professional organisation for those involved in the education and training of medical students and doctors. www.medicaleducators.org

CHAPTER 7
Introducing narrative reflection

Kathy Feest
Severn Deanery; UK Foundation Programme Office, Bristol, UK

Attending to one patient, one person at a time, one story at a time, is the material of narrative reflection. The lessons of humanity are located in the particular, and each story brings with it the seeds of learning. Reflective narrative is a powerful tool for clinicians and is easily available to all.

The Foundation Programme Learning Portfolio includes a section (3.1) entitled: 'Reflective practice: learning from experience'. The section begins by stating that, 'Good reflective practice is a core part of any learning programme' [1]. However, educational supervisors and their trainees often require a deeper understanding of what reflection is or can be in order to fully benefit from this aspect of their learning. Without further information, educational supervisors and their trainees are often baffled by this section of the portfolio. Part of the problem is that they approach reflective practice with the same clinical precision and from the same theoretical premise as they tackle the rest of the learning portfolio.

The concept of 'good' reflective practice suggests that there is also 'bad' reflective practice. Given these potential judgemental polarities, it is not surprising that we hear many trainees do not like the notion of reflection. They are not comfortable with the concept, and many sadly have come to think of reflection as a jargon word that has nothing to do with their experience of clinical practice or with them. For some trainees, reflection is reduced to an exercise of 'filling in the boxes' in order to be seen to have completed the necessary forms en route to successfully being signed off at the end of the year. Others, however, embrace the concept. Those who do, appreciate that reflection complements and extends their understanding and experience of both clinical practice and themselves. They recognise the personal and professional rewards that emerge from working with the raw material

Essential Guide to Educational Supervision in Postgraduate Medical Education, 1st edition. Edited by Nicola Cooper and Kirsty Forrest. © 2009 Blackwell Publishing, ISBN: 978-1-4051-7071-0.

of their experience as they endeavour to know more about their practice and themselves.

A reflective narrative account as a brief retelling of an event from clinical practice can result in important new understandings about the original event. Further, and importantly, this new narrative knowledge can then become embedded in the trainees' professional approach in future practice. Doctors who do not have enough time to engage with each meaningful situation they encounter during their busy clinical settings are often able to achieve a deeper understanding of situations when they choose to write about them later. Importantly the narrative thinking developed away from the clinical setting can begin to impose positively on the clinical setting itself.

Increasing trainees' understanding of how to employ narrative in this way could enable them to gain important insights into the heart of their practice – and themselves. It is also possible that those trainees who dislike the idea of written reflection also dislike getting too close to identifying the problems inherent in the nature of the medical encounter.

This chapter begins by briefly reviewing the competing premises that underpin the paradigms inherent in medical education. By viewing medicine as an interpretive event it is concluded that synthesis of a clinician's scientific acumen and human values is required in order to achieve the best outcomes with his or her patients. The chapter explores how doctors can employ their own experiences in service to their patients and themselves. It reframes the notion of reflection in an inclusive form that is accessible to both trainees and their supervisors. It ends by sharing one reflective narrative from practice that illustrates the previous theoretical discussion.

Where did 'reflection' come from?

Many educational supervisors may be more familiar with and indeed expect to engage with concepts that emerge from the 'positivist' paradigm. Fundamental to all positivist inquiry is the notion of the scientific presumption of truth. This primary principle of the positivist paradigm asserts that there is a reality that can be discovered, and is characterized by an epistemology that claims 'truth' for its findings [2–5]. This view of the world prioritises the collection of 'facts' over reflection and theoretical enquiry [6]. This positivist paradigm underpins the natural sciences model on which so much of good medicine is based. The quantitative nature of positivism includes the familiar '$n=x$' as a necessary component of much vital medical research and thinking.

However, the positivist paradigm of the natural sciences is not the only concept of value to postgraduate medical educators or their trainees. Another component of clinical education is firmly based in the social experiences of trainees as they learn to become professionals, and is expressed in words rather than in numbers. In this *qualitative* paradigm, things are viewed in their natural settings and practitioners endeavour to make sense of what they see by paying attention to the meanings people give to their social encounters. In the clinical setting the paradigm involves making sense of the lives and experiences of patients and their families, colleagues and other healthcare professionals. 'Making sense' is one of the distinguishing factors of qualitative research and this practice implies interpretation; hence, it is most often called 'interpretive inquiry'. 'Naturalistic studies', 'interpretive inquiries' or 'qualitative research' are phrases often used interchangeably to denote a qualitative paradigm [7,8].

A trainee's approach to creating meaning and understanding in his or her job is often linked to the ability to reflect and learn from those experiences that are expressed in qualitative rather than quantitative ways. As trainees work within hospital institutions with responsibility for patients, they are sometimes met with bewildering practices that do not equate either with the educational theory delivered in medical school or with familiar patterns of behaviour from colleagues or patients. Narrative reflection is one form of representation that enables the exploration of meaning as a social process. It emerges from the day-to-day experiential professional practice of trainees.

Reflection becomes the method of accessing and reassessing experiences in order to come to new conclusions or affirm suppositions that were just out of reach. Unlike so many material diagnostic tools of the doctors' trade, the experiential realm does not have a substance or object, or a material body on which to focus attention. Comprehension of ways of knowing and understanding these experiences can only be pursued in words. There is no comforting '$n=...$' anywhere to be seen. No surety or exact diagnosis is available. No wonder that so many professionals trained within a positivistic paradigm are sometimes uncomfortable with all these messy words. Explicitly articulating stories is a way of understanding both self and others involved in the same story. The learner both asks the questions and discovers the answers. In order to become effective professionals, trainee doctors require the knowledge inherent in both paradigms.

A narrative account both situates experience and frees the representation of that experience for those participating in it as readers and experiencers of the account. There is neither a singular 'right' answer to the questions at hand nor one 'right' question. By providing multiple interpretations of meaning, narrative knowing does not include the search for the grand narrative or one truth. Narrative meanings are not governed by the provision of quantifiable proof [9].

Reflection according to Schön

As in most professions relying on specialised knowledge, competence develops with experience and trainees' ability to construct solutions from the problems they are presented with develops through practice [10–12]. A crucial component to the early postgraduate years is learning through experience, or in Schön's term *learning in action* [10,13]. It is in the act of doing, within the experience itself, where discoveries about meaning take place.

Donald Schön made a great contribution to education when he identified how professionals learn [14]. The concepts of reflection-in-action and
reflection-on-action were central to Schön's work. Reflection-in-action is
often described as 'thinking on our feet'. It entails considering our experiences, connecting with our feelings and aligning them to the theories that
underpin our practice. These ideas are irreducible. It requires forming different views that then inform how we respond to the current evolving circumstances before us.

The professional can become perplexed or baffled, surprised or confused,
by new and unique experiences. He considers the situation based on his
previous thinking. He adjusts his thinking and changes the situation based
on the new information available to him [14]. This adjustment enables professionals to view each case as unique while drawing on the learning that
has occurred previously. This can then be associated to reflection-on-action,
which occurs later after the situation has passed.

In reflection-on-action, professionals use the tools of reflection in order
to reconsider and learn from their experiences. They may write down their
encounters, or talk them through with a colleague or a senior. This act of
reflection enables professionals to develop as they continuingly question
their approach and responses to their previous understanding of a situation.
It enables them to further refine the series of images, thoughts, examples,
cases and notions that they can draw upon to extend their knowledge. This
process of adding to their understanding and adjustment to their theories
about how things are is crucial to reflective thinking. Whenever professionals congregate they discuss and reflect on the current state of their profession. Doctors tell each other stories about patients, about fellow professionals
and about their hopes and dreams for their professional future. Reflection is
implicit in their growth as professionals. Educating young professional doctors means helping trainees to learn about the scientific basis of their clinical
world. It also means helping them to appreciate what it means to engage
within the human context of their professional world. Narrative reflection is
a means of helping them to do this.

What are we trying to achieve?

As emerging professionals, trainees must cope with the reality of what it
means for them to put their academic work into practice in the very human
sphere of medicine. That trainees must become technically adept and clin-
ically competent is undisputable. What is less articulated is the need for doctors to learn *how* to achieve all that their patients may reasonably want and
expect of them. Patients want doctors who possess more than the appropriate clinical acumen – they want doctors 'who comprehend what they go
through and who as a result stay the course with them through their illnesses. A medicine practiced without a genuine and obligating awareness
of what patients go through may fulfil its technical goals but it is an empty
medicine or at best, half a medicine' [15].

It is not possible for medical educators to demand trainees deal with each patient with compassion. No professional group can demand of its practitioners that they must become competent as human beings before they begin to practice their chosen profession. There are no easily identifiable '$n=...$' scales for measuring the qualities of a doctor. However, we all know when we are in the company of someone who listens to us and does not diminish our experiences or our telling of the event that brought us together in the first place. As practicing doctors, these people willingly listen to and engage with stories of illness that include both the clinical and the human dimensions.

Narrative reflection

Narrative is the primary means by which communities of practice transmit implicit knowledge such as norms, values, concepts and expectations [13]. Novices learn by interpreting narratives acquired within their community to form a personal 'manual of knowledge'. Narratives supply the conceptual scaffolding for understanding, interpreting and negotiating a community's way of knowing.

Reflections or written narrative accounts are situated both in the 'scientific' realm, where rigour and validity are the supreme determinants of precise acuity, and in the 'human' realm, where narrative knowing provides windows of understanding into the meanings that matter to an individual and to their society. These distinctions are also present in the medical model, and reflected in the process of writing reflective narratives.

Narrative moves us in some way because narrative has the capacity to mobilise our consciousness and feelings. Narrative helps us to identify what it is to be human. Narrative can draw our attention to our own moral code and has the capacity to call us to a moral awakening. This distinctive feature of narrative occurs because narratives are never value neutral but instead are revelatory. Embedded within the narrative are values that touch us. They enable us to consider the significance our community or society places on human life [16].

In questioning the lived experiences presented in narrative, we question the values of the people we meet in their particularised narrative experiences. We also question our own moral positions in relation to the narrative lives of the people we encounter. In our response to the lived experience of others we can reassess our own lived experience. We can then 'articulate and bring to language and awareness the narratives that we have developed to give meaning to our own lives' [9]. Through this reflective process of awareness we can reinterpret the events of the experiences we share through narrative and make changes in our own lives in our own practice.

The transformative nature of narrative means that through our interpretations of narrative it is possible for us to reinterpret it as we share the lived experiences and re-experience the lived experience as writers and readers and listeners of narrative accounts. We have the capacity to generate change so that new narratives can be recreated and re-emerged from our personal and collective interpretations [17].

Through their own reflective narrative accounts trainees can consider the themes embedded in these lived experiences secure in the knowledge that there are no 'right' answers to the questions that the narratives prompt. Instead, as educational tools they are presented as a means of providing questions that as tomorrow's doctors the trainees will need to consider for themselves and for their community.

Narrative prompts a kind of transferable skill across boundaries and helps people to interpret, co-operate, as well as convey their needs within their communities of practice. Because we use stories to learn about our situated culture and its practices, understanding narrative helps to increase the ability to recognise the rules for participation within our particular community of practice. This understanding also helps novices to interpret the expectations that will enable them to create a sense of belonging.

As they embark on their professional practice, trainees can begin to consider what it means to discharge their authority in practice. In preparing for their becoming the authors of their professional lives within the institutions where their practice will take place, narrative can help trainees to reconsider the issues that they have encountered.

Incorporating reflective narrative accounts in the experience of trainees' practice provides a dimension of professional inclusivity as well as a means of personal discovery. Personal reflection enables trainees to reconsider the professional and personal human challenges that they have met in practice.

The narrative reflections developed from practice contain stories that are current indicators of the cultural climate that doctors as well as their patients and colleagues meet in practice. Doctors who are able to consider and reflect on their own retold stories of lived experience can establish the moral imperatives that they might meet in future practice, as well as reconsider how to manage the situations that give rise to these experiences.

Trainee experiences raise questions relating to the value placed on human dignity, the definition of the person and the rights of the individual. The impact of the hierarchy of medicine and the adherence to the authority embedded within the hierarchy become individually and socially meaningful issues when anchored to a representation of that experience from practice.

Because meaning matters to humans, reflective narrative accounts not only represent the meaningful circumstances of a particular individual's lived experience but also convey the meaningful responses to the cultural circumstances provided by that experience. However, this situated and particular account in the final analysis cannot belong exclusively to the individual because the interpretation is developed from a shared social process. Meaning is not discovered like a new strain of a virus but is discovered through our representations, which are then shared [18].

Although narratives are partial representations and not the total experience, they enable us to question the multiple layers of the meaning of the experience itself. As readers or listeners of the experience, we may come to a different interpretation than that proffered by the writer or teller of the account. Our concerns about the experiences may indeed be different than those posited by the narrative's author. Trainee doctors, educational supervisors, nurses, medical administrators, chief executives, patients and loved ones will all bring a dimension to the narrative that is unique to their particular perspective. Consequently, sharing narratives within a community of practice extends the meanings and shared understandings of the experience itself. Sharing narrative reflections can become a building block of the professional's community of practice.

The reflective narrative tool box

Reflective narrative writing is a tool that enables its practitioners to access levels of meaning that otherwise can be left unresolved. Making a scene fictional – what narrative writing achieves – involves creating characters as a way of making them real. The reflections on the page detail situations and events that involve participants. The clinical scenarios that are described are those that sit at the edge of memory and somehow continue to need to be processed. These reflections that emerge from the tip of the pen unannounced often reveal the most promising self-revelatory dimensions. The stories we tell in written reflections are those where lessons remain to be learned.

Written reflection can be a powerful method for reframing and reshaping events. Doctors are regularly called upon to tell and then witness the result of telling painful truths. Stories that cannot easily be borne by the patient are often shared exclusively with the doctor and other members of the healthcare team. As witnesses of the stories they retell, revelations about their place in the story may change. Trainees may see that they have written a story precisely because they were the witness for their patients, or colleagues. Retelling a story releases the burden of exclusivity on the witness of the events.

One of the dilemmas of being a doctor is being left to become one's own judge of a situation one finds oneself in. Writing a story about a clinical encounter in which one was once a main character creates a place where it is possible to witness the events and review them differently. Accessing new levels of understanding from the narrative can become a powerful way of learning and synthesising the experience of practice. Learning in this way respects a doctor's own identity and ability to discover new ways of thinking. It reinforces and reviews the values that enable the continuing and ongoing quest for the improvement required of professionals.

Doctors are experienced writers. Every day they write remarks in their patients' notes, and write letters to each other and to patients to convey treatment options or plans. These structured writings allow little of the doctors' voice. Instead, they communicate meaning in a technologically efficient manner. There is no room for communicating what it is like to empathise with a patient or his family, and no place to disclose the rage that was felt after the death of a patient that particularly moved them. The experience of these meaningful aspects of medicine shape the future practice of professionals and it is these moments that require attention.

Giving permission to trainees to write about their experiences, thoughts, feelings, values and concerns is one way of enabling them to create a process of meaningful engagement with their clinical world. Writing enables trainees to access their interior world and pose questions through examples of practice that can then illuminate their clinical world and help them make sense of their own lives.

Professor Rita Charon gives a simple yet effective model for giving permission to trainees to write reflective accounts. She tells her students:

'Every day you write in the hospital chart (notes) about each of your patients. You know exactly what to write there and the form in which to write it. You write about your patient's current complaints, the results of the physical exam, laboratory findings, opinions of consultants and the plan. If your patient dying of prostate cancer reminds you of your grandfather, who died of that disease last summer, and each time you go into the patients' room, you weep for your grandfather, you can not write that in the notes. We will not let you. And yet it has to be written somewhere. You write it in the Parallel Chart'. [15]

She tells students that the writing is indexed to a particular patient. It is neither a diary nor a letter. Neither is it a general examination of one's life. Instead, it is 'narrative writing in the service of the care of a particular patient'.

These distinctions are in contrast to many writers who have prepared step by step 'how to do it' models of reflection [19–21]. These usually suggest that reflection can be achieved in a neat linear sequence. This immediately encourages the technical reductionist view of the exercise and misses the point. The legacy of the positivist approach then stifles the interior journey. Instead, the Charon approach gives permission for trainees to be involved in their own clinical experiences. This approach connects with the nature of the interpretative paradigm where meaning matters. This type of reflection is meaningful and powerful. The first step is giving permission for it to occur. Contrast this instruction with the learning portfolios: 'Try to put time aside each day to reflect on the day's learning opportunities and identify any further learning needs.' Giving permission to be human and connected to a patient is central to reflective writing. The learning will then emerge from the example that the trainee has used.

Practitioners need to learn how to pay attention to those experiences that are meaningful to them and why this is so. Sharing the results of their narrative reflections with educational supervisors, or other colleagues, is an important component on the journey of becoming professionals.

Writing reflections without sharing them is like cooking a good meal and not eating it. The ingredients are assembled, prepared and presented but no health-giving properties can occur until the food is eaten and digested. Eating alone nourishes but is rarely as satisfying as having a meal with another person. The benefits of narrative writing are similar. It is better to eat alone than starve, but when shared, narrative writing becomes food for the soul.

Viewed as part of clinical training when shared with educational supervisors, the narrative reflections take their place in mainstream medical education and are not viewed as a marginal activity by the trainees. The trainees are then able to become the authors of their professional lives with permission to learn from and engage with their patients.

Narrative reflection in practice

Reading trainees' as well as medical students' work is a powerful and rewarding way of learning about narrative reflection for trainees and educational supervisors alike. The following is a reflective narrative that was written by a medical student as an undergraduate assignment. The set task was to write about an experience that occurred during the shadowing component of the final-year course. It beautifully illustrates and synthesises many of the issues that have been discussed earlier in the text. There is no right or wrong, or good or bad interpretation of this work. It is presented in its complete form and offers the reader an opportunity to share an individual clinical experience. It is only one story of the many that could be told. Yet it is here in the individual's story, the witnessed narrative, where the experiences of learning emerge.

Life can change in a second.
Life can change in a second; meeting the man of your dreams, meeting another car head on, meeting your breaker of bad news on the morning ward round. We can never know what lies just around the corner. As a medical student, I have frequently seen doctors telling patients bad news, and I have always felt privileged to be present, yet almost voyeuristic; nothing more than a silent, sympathetic, staring witness. I have always felt sad for the patients, but detached. During my shadowing week, I found myself unexpectedly affected by seeing a patient being told she had inoperable bowel cancer.

She was sitting up in bed. Her cheeks were hollow, her hair limp and tired. There was no sparkle in her eyes, no flesh on her desperately thin frame. She smiled at us, looking for signs of hope, for good news, for any clues from our body language as to what was coming next. I drew the curtains round as we lined up as if for battle; doctors versus relatives, patient in the middle, nurse hovering between factions to ensure fair play. Her father stood next to her, but he was too old now to keep his daughter out of harm's way. Her husband was her guardian angel, standing at the foot of the bed; out of eye contact with everyone except his beautiful wife.

'We have failed this patient' was my only thought. She had presented over 15 months ago with bowel symptoms, and was fully investigated. How had her cancer not been found? Somehow, I felt as though I was personally responsible. She was only 51; my mother's age.

All eyes were on the consultant. What would he say? He was gentle, clear, genuine and faultless in his delivery. Brilliant, in fact, given the circumstances. He had not removed the tumour, he said; it would have been too big an operation for her in her current frail state. He said that the cancer was not just in the bowel; the tumour had stuck her bowel to her uterus, and had spread to her liver and both sides of her diaphragm. He wished he could have been standing there telling her that he'd removed all the cancer, he said, but all he had done was to bypass it. He had not removed anything at all.

I didn't know where to look. I realised my heart was pounding and my eyes were welling up. She never moved her gaze from the bearer of bad news; her angel of death. Her life had changed in a second. Was she still listening to him? How could she take all this in? 'Advanced cancer...', 'Extensive disease...', 'Some chemotherapy might help...', 'The oncologist will come and see you...', 'I wish I was standing here telling you that I have removed all the cancer...'.

I looked around the characters in this scene, putting myself into each person's shoes in turn. How was the patient so gentle and accepting? Why wasn't she angry? Her husband stared at the floor. I looked at her father who was looking at me. I saw no anger, no disbelief, no blame, just deep sadness and grave understanding in his eyes. Should I look down, look away, smile one of those hopeless half-smiles of pity? Was he looking for a glimmer of hope in my eyes, trying to shake himself out of this bad dream? I held his gaze a moment longer, and then he looked back to his daughter. Is it true that the eye is the window to the soul? Could he see my genuine sadness, coming from that part of the heart so deep that it must actually be in the stomach, because it was making me feel sick. His daughter was the same age as my mother. I tried not to let my imagination rewrite the scene with a different character playing the lead.

I was clutching the patient's notes, but scribbling, 'Obs stable, apyrexial, patient not in pain, diagnosis explained, husband and father present', seemed rather a callous oversimplification of the situation. How could I write, 'Re-site cannula, phone oncologist, refer to dietician,' on the jobs list, while this lady was trying to imagine how long she had left in this world? I would write later.

We seemed to be in the cubicle forever – the medical trio and the family trio – staring at each other. Finally, the full, unabridged version of the bad news had been broken. The patient had nodded, smiled gently, said, 'Yes' throughout. She looked so thin, so vulnerable, so helpless. The consultant asked if she had any questions.

'Will I be able to go home again at all?' asked the patient. 'Will I die here in hospital?' was what she was really asking. When she heard she should be well enough to go home and could have chemotherapy as an outpatient, she beamed a smile so radiant that her eyes almost twinkled.

How had she readjusted so fast? She had been hoping to hear that all her tumour had been removed; she was told it had spread everywhere. But there was no anger, no blame, no recriminations, no tears; not yet, anyway. Just a dazzling smile across her pale, thin face when she heard that the end was not here and now; she would be able to go home. How had she reset her expectations of life so quickly?

We left the curtains closed to protect the shell shocked trio. The father and husband powerless now to protect this woman whom they loved so deeply. What words of comfort would they find to offer each other now that their lives had been turned upside down in a few seconds? Were the magic curtains containing the conversation from the other three patients in the bay?

Were they thanking their lucky stars it wasn't them? Would they know what to say when the curtains were opened again?

Post script
Her condition deteriorated and she was taken to ICU two days after I wrote this. I found myself going there everyday to see how she was doing, until I realised that she was never going to go home again, and then I couldn't bear to go anymore.

The 'learning need' to be developed in my PRHO year would be to maintain perfect poise on the knife-edge between emotional involvement and professional detachment. Fortunately, however, most of us are human beings, not machines, and falling either way is inevitable and acceptable. It is important, from an emotional survival point of view, to try and predict which patients affect us most, and not to fall too far … and also, not to feel personally guilty for things which cannot be changed.

I can still hear her hopeful little voice, 'I was hoping you were going to say you'd taken it all out'. And I can still see her brave, dazzling smile at the thought of going home [22].

Your turn
This chapter ends by extending an invitation to you to pick up a pen and write one short account from your practice. It will not take long, probably less time than it took to read this chapter. Given permission to write a tale from your clinical experience, what will you write about? Will you willingly share that experience with your trainee when they next ask what this thing called 'reflection' is all about?

References

1. The Department of Health, Foundation Programme learning portfolio. http://www.foundationprogramme.nhs.uk/.
2. Harris RW. Absolutism and enlightenment. Blandford, London, 1967.
3. Kuhn TS. The structure of scientific revolutions. University of Chicago Press, London, 1970.

4. Kleinman A. Writing at the margin. University of California Press, London, 1995.
5. Popper KR. The logic of scientific discovery. Hutchinson & Co. (Publishers) Ltd., London, 1962.
6. Marshall G. Dictionary of sociology. Oxford University Press, Oxford, New York, 1998.
7. Denzin NK, Lincoln Y (Eds). Handbook of qualitative research. Sage, London, Thousand Oaks, New Delhi, 2000.
8. Lincoln Y. Emerging criteria for quality in qualitative and interpretive research. *Qual Inq* 1995; **1 (3)**: 275–289.
9. Polkinghorne DE. Narrative knowing and the human sciences. State University of New York Press, Albany, New York, 1988.
10. Schön D. Educating the reflective practitioner. Jossey Bass, San Francisco, 1987.
11. Dilworth JP, Mitchell DM. Comparison of the views of junior doctors, consultants and managers on work and training. *J R Coll Physicians Lond* 1998; **32 (4)**: 344–350.
12. Ende J. Feedback in medical education. *J Am Med Assoc* 1983; **250**: 777–781.
13. Wenger E. Communities of practice learning meaning and identity. Cambridge University Press, Cambridge, 1999.
14. Schön D. The reflective practitioner. How professionals think in action. Arena, London, 1983.
15. Charon R. Narrative medicine honoring the stories of illness. Oxford University Press, Oxford, 2006.
16. Bruner J. The narrative construction of reality. *Crit Inq* 1991; **18**: 1–21.
17. Macintyre A. After virtue. Gerald Duckworth & Co. Ltd., London, 1981.
18. Bruner J. Acts of meaning. Harvard University Press, London, 1990.
19. Atkins S, Murphy K. Reflective practice. *Nurs Stand* 1994; **8 (39)**: 49–56.
20. Kolb DA. Experiential learning: experience as the source of learning and development. Prentice Hall, New Jersey, 1984.
21. Gibbs G. Learning by doing: a guide to teaching and learning methods. Oxford Further Education Unit, Oxford Brookes University, Oxford, 1988.
22. Feest K, Forbes K. Today's students tomorrow's doctors. Radcliffe Publishing, Oxford, 2006.

CHAPTER 8
Assessments and appraisal

Julian Archer
Peninsula College of Medicine and Dentistry, Plymouth, UK

This chapter focuses on the main work-based assessments used in postgraduate medical education programmes. These are underpinned by research and statistical evidence, some of which is described in order to help educational supervisors understand important concepts around assessment. The practicalities of work-based assessments and how to interpret the results are then discussed. Feedback is at the heart of every well-formulated assessment programme, so this is also described in some detail. Finally, this chapter looks briefly at appraisal, which is a complementary but different process with different aims.

Modernising medical careers (MMC) has been a fundamental change in postgraduate medical education. Part of this has been the development of foundation programmes [1]. One of the key aims of foundation programmes is that trainees are formally assessed with respect to their competency in defined areas of clinical practice within a curriculum [2], and central to its effectiveness is therefore a robust work-based assessment programme [3]. The Postgraduate Medical Education and Training Board (PMETB) approves and oversees each programme and initially focuses on three of its nine key assessment principles [4], as highlighted in Box 8.1. This has put the need to evaluate and quality assure assessment methods and programmes at the heart of postgraduate medical education for the first time.

In order to explore the purpose of any assessment programme, it is important to first define some key terms and concepts in current assessment thinking.

Key concepts in assessment

Assessment is a process in which explicit measurements and judgements are made against defined (usually external) criteria [5]. This is very different from appraisal in which performance is under review but the criteria against

Essential Guide to Educational Supervision in Postgraduate Medical Education, 1st edition. Edited by Nicola Cooper and Kirsty Forrest. © 2009 Blackwell Publishing, ISBN: 978-1-4051-7071-0.

Box 8.1 PMETB assessment principles

- The assessment system must be fit for a range of purposes*.
- Content of the assessment must be based on curricula referenced to *Good Medical Practice**.
- Methods used will be selected in the light of purpose and content of that component of the assessment programme.
- Methods used to set standards for trainees' competence must be transparent and in the public domain.
- Assessments must provide relevant feedback*.
- Assessors/examiners will be recruited against criteria for performing the tasks they undertake.
- There will be lay input into the development of assessment.
- Documentation will be standardised and made accessible nationally.
- There will be resources sufficient to support assessment.

* indicates the three principles highlighted by PMETB.

which this is undertaken are usually individual and internalised, and the process is confidential, reflective and supportive.

Purpose

A clear definition of the purpose and object of assessment is important in selecting the appropriate method. This is particularly relevant because assessment drives learning [6], so it is fundamental that assessment is appropriate and proportionate. Having determined what it is that one needs to measure, one must ask several further questions. For example, should the assessment be formative or summative?

Formative assessment is characterised by an interest in personal development. The outcome measures are primarily used by an individual for personal development planning. The performance is internally evaluated, perhaps with external comparative data, but not used to make a definitive judgement. Summative assessment can be defined as a measurement of an individual compared to a norm or criterion referenced standard, from which a decision about the individual is made. (Norm referencing describes an individual's performance in terms of his or her position in a group; criterion referencing describes whether an individual achieved a certain score.)

However, current trends challenge this traditional separatist view [7]. It is argued that well formulated and correctly implemented 'summative' assessment can not only provide decisive measurements but also provide structured 'formative' feedback to support professional development. In this way assessment outputs can inform appraisal processes but appraisal outcomes does not inform assessment.

The role of assessment in postgraduate medical education

Assessment programmes in postgraduate medical education have been developed in order to:
- provide feedback to trainees to help them improve;
- meet the PMETB assessment principles (quality assurance);
- determine whether a trainee is fit to progress to the next stage of training;
- identify doctors who may be in difficulty.

Assessment tools can and should be designed to generate feedback as well as identify poor performers. This is often described as a quality improvement model, where focussed feedback is provided to participants with the aim of improving their overall performance, both those who are doing well and those about whom concerns are raised [8]. A balance has to be achieved between delivering robust assessments and informing personal development.

There is a tendency to use formative assessment as an excuse for poorly performed assessment. The relative importance of assessment characteristics will vary depending on the intended purpose [9], but the basic principles of assessment methodology should be adhered to for both formative and summative assessments. Having defined the focus of any assessment, we must evaluate the method to ensure that it will carry out its purpose. This is undertaken by exploring a number of concepts, starting with validity.

Validity

Validity is whether or not an assessment measures what it is supposed to measure. A particular assessment might be valid for one purpose but not for another. However, it is more complicated than that [10]. There is no single measure of validity, and it is not an all-or-nothing concept. There are five main 'types' of validity, shown in Box 8.2 [11,12]. Validity has also been

Box 8.2

The main 'types' of validity

Type	Definition
Face	Looks as though it measures what is intended
Content	The extent to which an assessment measures the intended content area, for example an assessment derived from mapping to a curriculum
Construct	The extent to which an assessment measures a hypothetical construct, for example reasoning skills Domain theory: tasks, attitudes or behaviours are chosen because they are believed to be part of the same construct, and not related to another area (domain), for example professionalism
Criterion	The extent to which the scores are related to concrete criteria
Predictive	The degree to which an assessment predicts future performance

described as 'evidence ... to support or refute the meaning or interpretation assigned to assessment results' [13]. What an assessment result means to individuals or groups *across settings or contexts* is an ongoing question, which is why validity is an evolving concept and validation a continuing process.

Reliability

Reliability is the degree to which a test *consistently* measures whatever it measures. It can be defined as the reproducibility of assessment results over time or different occasions. In science, the ability to reproduce an experiment's findings is fundamental. Three approaches to reliability are briefly discussed: internal consistency, classical theory and generalisability (G) theory [14].

Internal consistency

Internal consistency is also known as test–retest reliability. A repeated test to the same group of candidates should produce the same result. Internal consistency can be measured using Cronbach's alpha [15]. Cronbach's alpha can be applied to the consistency among items in a test as well as to the stability of performance scores on multiple trials of the same test. This is used in providing evidence for the reliability of the rating scale, but is of limited value in performance assessment where inter-rater consistency (i.e. the differences between assessor perception of performance) is often the most significant confounding factor.

Classical theory

In classical theory it is the true difference between individuals, assuming one exists, which is of interest, and not a difference that is attributable to an external factor, for example an assessor who consistently gives low marks (a hawk). True score is conceptualised as the average score a person would achieve if assessed an infinitely large number of times. The difference between the observed score and the true score is the measurement error. The relevance of this will be seen when we look at the different work-based assessments.

Reliability is traditionally estimated by evaluating one source of potential error at a time.

- *Inter-rater reliability*
  Assessors often vary in their interpretation of an event, even if they are assessing the same candidate at the same time (this can be estimated using the kappa statistic).
- *Intra-rater reliability*
  Assessors are sometimes not consistent within themselves when rating from one event to another.
- *Case specificity*
  Professional performance is complicated by the nature of the problem being faced. Explaining a medical diagnosis to a patient might be performed well if it is a certain diagnosis and a certain patient, but badly with a different diagnosis or an angry patient. So one case will not necessarily generalise to the 'universe' of cases and patients.

However, evaluating one source of potential error at a time is often impractical and inaccurate. Generalisability theory attempts to overcome this.

Generalisability (G) theory

Generalisability theory is a statistical method used to estimate variance for all the variables of interest in an assessment. It allows key sources of error to be quantified without multiple experiments [14]. It is used in analysing reliability for undergraduate and postgraduate examinations. The G coefficient, which represents the reliability of an actual sample, can be used to predict reliability if one facet of the assessment were to be modified, for example the number of cases or question items. This can be used to increase reliability to an acceptable level, although reliability should always then be re-evaluated.

Feasibility

Feasibility refers to practicality. To achieve the ultimate in reliability and validity, an individual should be assessed by an infinite number of assessors in an infinite number of cases. This is obviously not feasible. The statistical modelling described in the previous paragraph is used within the constraints of *practicality* to achieve validity and reliability [9].

Feasibility can be explored in a number of ways including the time taken and personnel needed to administer, collate and feedback results, as well as costs and response rates. The work-based assessments used in postgraduate medical education have all been evaluated in terms of their feasibility.

The foundation assessment programme

Taking the foundation programme as an example, in 2003 several deaneries collaborated in a pilot programme across the UK to establish the feasibility of an assessment programme and to gather preliminary data about the performance of the assessment tools and the educational impact on trainees.

When developing any assessment programme, there are some key considerations:

- clarifying the purpose;
- mapping the assessments to the curriculum;
- determining validity, reliability and feasibility;
- determining the educational impact.

In addition, an increasing body of evidence is available from existing assessment programmes, for example for residency programmes in the United States. A pragmatic approach was also required with regard to the curriculum. It would only be feasible to assess core components of it.

In most part of England and Wales, the work-based assessments used in the foundation programmes are:

- mini-CEX (clinical evaluation exercise);
- DOPS (direct observation of procedural skills);
- 360° feedback – also known as 'mini-PAT' (peer assessment tool) or TAB (team assessment of behaviours);
- CbD (case-based discussion).

In Scotland, the assessments used are:
- presented evidence, including a reflective portfolio and personal development plan;
- workplace assessment of the skills listed in the foundation curriculum;
- 360° feedback;
- educational supervisor's report.

Box 8.3 summarises the four assessment instruments used in England and Wales. They were either chosen from existing assessment programmes in

---

Box 8.3

Assessment instruments used in England and Wales

Type of assessment instrument	Summary	Setting	Time required (median)
Mini-CEX	Assessment of whole or part of an actual clinical encounter (three parts – history, examination and counselling) 7 questions and global rating scale	Focus on acute care • Emergency Department • Post-take ward round • Home visit	25 min
DOPS	Assessment of whole or part of an actual technical procedure 11 questions and global rating scale	Daily and on-call work	15 min
360° feedback	Feedback from a range of co-workers across the domains of *Good Medical Practice* which includes both clinical and professional attributes Mini-PAT: 14 questions and global rating scale TAB: 4 global questions	Any clinical setting (although more challenging with less exposure to a clinical team, e.g. general practice, or less clinical exposure, e.g. pathology)	Each assessor 7 min
CBD	Assessment based on discussion arising from a trainee's entry in the notes. This attempts to measure clinical reasoning 7 questions and global rating scale	Pre-arranged office setting	25 min

postgraduate medical education or developed specifically to assess a range of foundation competencies.

Face-to-face training of assessors in how to use the assessment instruments is extremely important in order to maximise validity and reliability. Training includes:

- observation training (how to observe, the forms used);
- performance dimension training (whether assessing knowledge, skills, clinical judgement or professionalism);
- frame of reference training (the agreed acceptable standard for the level of doctor being observed).

Problems observed during research include assessors who do not actually observe, are too lenient or too harsh, do not discriminate the performance of a trainee across different domains, or may not themselves possess the skills which they are observing.

Mini-CEX and DOPS

The mini-CEX was already well established by the American Board of Internal Medicine as a way of assessing clinical skills [16]. Assessors observe a 'snapshot' of a clinical encounter. The instrument was anglicised prior to piloting in the UK. In a similar way, DOPS had already been piloted by the Royal College of Physicians of London [17].

360° feedback

The use of 360° (or multisource) feedback to assess aspects of Good Medical Practice [18] was already established in the UK. The Sheffield Peer Review Assessment Tool (SPRAT) [19] was analysed and adapted for use in the foundation programmes, and it became mini-PAT [20]. Its initial validity was established using a range of statistical methods, and its contents were mapped against the foundation curriculum.

CbD

The ability of chart stimulated recall or case-based discussion to investigate doctors' decision-making led to its widespread introduction to assess doctors in Canada and the United States [21]. Clinical reasoning is a key part of clinical performance. CbD uses the doctor and his notes to get a fuller picture of the case and provides additional information that is rarely discerned through record review alone. CbD in the foundation programme was built on international literature on this subject and work undertaken as part of the General Medical Council's performance review procedures [22].

Establishing a rating scale

The rating scales for the foundation programme assessments were established after an extensive literature review. All types of rating formats are subject to cognitive processing distortions [23]; that is, assessors do not simply report what they have observed. A numerical scale providing a continuum is fundamental [24], with clear descriptions to define the scale in order to support reliability [25]. Much of the literature centres on the suitability of a 5- to 9-point scale [26], with further evidence for the use of an even number [27].

Making the decision: synthesising work-based assessment evidence

Understanding how each component of an assessment programme fits into the overall picture is important. It is essential that all work-based assessments of a trainee are reviewed and any developmental needs identified. An *assessment profile* is required to determine whether the performance of a trainee is satisfactory or not. Profiling relies on the triangulation of work-based assessment evidence [28], followed by an expert judgement based on it. The expert judgement lies, in the first instance, with the educational supervisor.

The evidence in most assessment programmes contains both quantitative (scores) and qualitative (free text) information, enhancing the value of overall judgements by providing a richness of data. Evaluation of a portfolio will increasingly be central in the decision-making process, but it must be remembered that a portfolio is only as good as its parts.

The following criteria must all be satisfied to identify the clearly satisfactory trainee:
- Timely submission of all the required work-based assessments *with appropriate sampling across the required clinical content as well as assessors.*
- Evidence of remediation of any earlier identified development needs.
- No concerns should have been raised in relation to probity or fraud.

The following criteria would each individually constitute unsatisfactory performance:
- failure to participate in a work-based assessment (other than when prevented from doing so by the nature of the post, ill health or other approved leave);
- failure to reach the expected standard for their stage of training for all the required work-based assessments;
- failure to remediate developmental needs despite an agreed and appropriately supported action plan;
- any evidence of fraud.

What do I do if I am not sure whether the performance of a trainee is satisfactory or not?

The minimum number of assessments required in the foundation programme is based on the confidence we can apply to the overall outcome (see Box 8.4). For the majority of trainees their aggregated score can be placed confidently on one side or the other of the satisfactory/unsatisfactory cut-off. However, a borderline trainee may need more assessments. The assessment programme is designed to help focus more assessments on those trainees who need them. Additional assessments can be used to describe the nature of the problem(s) more clearly. These additional assessments can be either standard foundation assessments and/or alternative assessments.

Box 8.4

The 95% CI to be placed around a trainee mean score for the number of assessors contributing to that score

	Mini-CEX	DOPS	Mini-PAT	CBD
4 cases	0.55	0.59	0.57	0.55
6 cases	0.45	0.48	0.47	0.45
8 cases	0.39	0.42	0.40	0.39
12 cases	0.32	0.34	0.33	0.32

There are a number of ways in which extra assessments will increase the robustness of the judgement being made. As the number of assessors increases, the confidence intervals (CIs) narrow. For example, for mini-CEX the 95% CI for 4 cases is 0.55 but for 12 cases is 0.32 on a 6-point scale where the cut-off score is taken as 4.0. In other words, an overall mean of 4.33 would represent a 'pass' if achieved with 12 cases (CI 4.02–4.64) but one could not be 95% confident that the individual had 'passed' with only 4 cases (CI 3.77–4.89).

Additional sampling will also allow a broader *qualitative* perspective on the trainees' performance, enabling a clearer understanding of the nature of the problem and providing additional opportunities to identify action points and remediation.

Where work-based assessments have raised concerns about a particular aspect of performance it may be appropriate to use alternative assessments to describe the problem in more detail. For example, if a trainee has had concerns raised about his communication with patients, then the use of video to record, assess and debrief the trainee's communication skills may be appropriate.

Feedback

What is the evidence that feedback matters?

In a recent best evidence medical education review looking at assessment, feedback and physicians' clinical performance [29], 41 studies were identified that fulfilled the inclusion criteria: performance of practising doctors in a clinical setting, not confounded by other interventions, and where the doctor was the centre of focus. The review concluded that feedback can positively change clinical performance when it is systematically delivered from credible sources.

It is clear that the relationship between the recipient [29] and the provision process [30], most notably the facilitation [31] and the nature of the feedback [32], contributes to the outcome for each individual participant. The recipient must feel in a position to accept the feedback, neither blaming others nor doubting the credibility of assessors [33]. The challenge appears to lie with those who receive negative feedback and the support required in dealing with this. Negative feedback does not have to have an entirely negative outcome but there is a risk.

Giving feedback

The provision of feedback has two components: the content and the process by which the content is delivered [34]. For feedback to be effective its content must be clear and understood by both subject and facilitator. Its delivery should be timely, interactive, face-to-face, and in a non-judgemental environment [35]. This is often not undertaken well in the clinical setting [36] where clinicians are reluctant to give negative feedback or fail failing doctors [37].

The final step and the focus of interest is in using feedback for learning and/or performance change. There is evidence that feedback from assessment processes can be positive for the individual and for an organisation [37,38]. However, there is also evidence that it can be a negative experience [32]. Evidence to date shows that some interventions appear more effective than others, and this is because medical practice and behaviour are influenced and changed by personal, professional and environmental factors.

It is easy to think of work-based assessments as burdensome, but it is important to remember the educational value of feedback. Feedback in the foundation programme is delivered in two main settings: in real time after case-focussed assessments, and when delivering collated feedback from 360° assessment tools. A useful model for feedback in postgraduate medical education is proposed by Holmboe *et al.* [33]:
- To be most effective, feedback needs to be *interactive* so that trainees can embrace and take ownership of their strengths and weaknesses.
- Self-assessment should be encouraged for effective reflection.
- An explicit action plan should be developed to 'close the loop' and focus on change.

How do I approach giving negative feedback?

It is important to ensure that the discussion focuses on areas of strength as well as areas in need of improvement. When possible, try and review other assessments or evidence that might be available.

For identifying the problem:
- give the trainees the opportunity to present their views first;
- clarify areas of concern;
- explore the trainees' insight into problem areas – whether they agree with concerns raised or not (try to use the evidence to help the trainees gain a better understanding of their performance);

- discuss whether problems are sufficiently clearly defined to be able to develop a remediation plan or whether more evidence is needed to help clarify the problem;
- consider whether there are factors outside work (distractors), for example home problems, stress or ill health that may be interfering with the trainees' ability to function well at work.

For addressing the problem and supporting the trainee:

- get the trainee to suggest ideas to address problem areas;
- set learning objectives and timescales for improvement, and document these in a personal development plan;
- suggest targeted training and feedback in the areas identified;
- agree ways in which more evidence might be collected when the problem is not clear, or where clarification of the nature of the problem is needed;
- discuss with the trainee ways in which you can support and help.

Exploring the trainee's insight into problem areas is a very important aspect of giving negative feedback. Kruger and Dunning found that incompetence causes not only poor performance but also the inability to recognise that one's performance is poor [39]. This was demonstrated in a series of experiments that showed that participants in the bottom quartile of performance not only overestimated themselves, but also thought they were above average (see Figure 8.1), whereas top performers underestimated themselves – a phenomenon

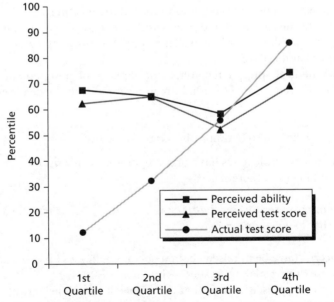

Figure 8.1 Perceived ability and test performance as a function of actual test performance. Also known as the 'Kruger–Dunning effect'.
Reproduced with permission Ref [39].

frequently observed in clinical practice. The same research suggested that one way to help people recognise their areas for development is to train them to be competent in the task in question. This is because, through training, 'they also gain the metacognitive skills to recognise the previous error of their ways'.

It can sometimes be helpful for the trainee to nominate a mentor who will identify when problem practice arises, so that any issues can be addressed immediately. Neutral support networks should be offered if appropriate, for example counselling services. The objectives should be recorded in the trainee's learning plan and reviewed after an appropriate time. This learning plan should be agreed and signed by both trainee and supervisor. In addition, a letter to the trainee following the meeting with the agreed plan provides a clear record of the discussion and its outcomes.

Trainees in serious difficulty

If a trainee is in serious difficulty (defined in Box 8.5), it is advisable prior to the meeting to:
- speak with appropriate colleague(s) about the trainee's feedback and agree where the problems are (try and ensure you have examples of specific behaviour to illustrate areas of concern);
- inform the trainee in advance that there are concerns with his or her feedback and give the opportunity to bring a mutually acceptable colleague to the meeting for support;
- have a short time interval between telling the trainees that there is a concern and meeting with them to discuss this;
- nominate someone to document minutes of the meeting;
- send the trainee a record of the discussion and agreed action plan after the meeting and ask him or her to sign a copy to confirming agreement with the record and actions.
- involve neutral support networks, the director of postgraduate medical education, occupational health, human resources and the deanery.

Box 8.5 Definition of a trainee in serious difficulty

- A number of colleagues have raised significant concerns over practice in a number of different areas
  or
- One or more serious incident(s) has been identified in which patient care has been compromised
  or
- Concerns have been raised about a doctor's ability to function safely because of personal difficulties including ill health

If the concerns raised suggest that the trainee is in serious difficulty, then the feedback and any other concerns should be discussed with the programme director and the director of postgraduate medical education.

The International Performance Assessment Coalition, a collaboration of international medical educationalists, has outlined a useful model for doctors who may require remedial training:
- identify where remediation should take place;
- decide on the time frame of the remediation;
- document goals and objectives;
- plan remedial programme;
- plan a date for re-assessment (and the nature of the assessment);
- decide on re-entry into practice following re-assessment;
- continue monitoring (if successfully remediated).

Appraisal

Annual appraisal for all doctors in the UK became a contractual obligation in 2001, and is now linked to revalidation that all career grade doctors will have to achieve every 5 years. The results of assessments (e.g. 360° feedback) often feed into the appraisal process. However, appraisal is an entirely different process with different aims.

Appraisal is designed to allow doctors time out to reflect on their performance in different areas. Appraisal is a process in which:
- performance in different clinical and non-clinical areas is reviewed, based on the GMC document *Good Medical Practice* [18] – see Box 8.6;
- professional roles and priorities are explored;
- progress on previously agreed objectives is reviewed;
- achievements are recognised;
- individual and organisational objectives are aligned;
- ways in which the organisation can help the individual make their best contribution are explored.

The last two points apply particularly to career grade doctors, in which appraisals are closely linked to job planning. For trainees, the emphasis is more on agreeing an *educational* personal development plan with some short- and long-term goals. This is done in light of a portfolio review, which includes the output from assessments.

Box 8.6 The different areas covered in *Good Medical Practice*

- Good clinical care
- Maintaining good medical practice (e.g. continuing professional development)
- Teaching and training
- Relationships with patients
- Working with colleagues (e.g. including results of 360° feedback)
- Probity and health

A key aspect of appraisal is that it is *confidential*. It should take place in private and without interruptions. The relationship between appraisee and appraiser should be one of trust and respect. If that is not the case, there should be flexibility in the system for an appraisee to choose another appraiser. It should also result in action points, or a personal development plan. The action points should be SMART, that is:

- Specific
- Measurable
- Attainable
- Realistic
- Timed

It is a normal practice to use standard documentation, although this varies depending on the doctor and the organisation involved. Appraisal is a process through which a doctor can develop his or her skills and career, and it can also be used by educational supervisors to set personal development plans related to their educational role.

References

1. Department of Health. Modernising Medical Careers, the next steps. The future shape of Foundation, specialist and general practice training programmes. DH, London, 2004. www.dh.gov.uk
2. Academy of Medical Royal Colleges and the Departments of Health. Foundation Programme Curriculum, 2007. www.foundationprogramme.nhs.uk
3. Davies H, Archer J, Heard S, Southgate L. Assessment tools for Foundation programmes – a practical guide. *BMJ Career Focus* 2005; **330**: 195–196.
4. Postgraduate Medical Education and Training Board. Principles for an assessment system for postgraduate medical training. PMETB, London, 2005.
5. Jolly B. Assessment and appraisal. *Med Educ* 1997; **31(Suppl. 1)**: 20–24.
6. Newble D, Jaeger K. The effects of assessments and examinations on the learning of medical students. *Med Educ* 1983; **17(3)**: 165–171.
7. Govaerts MJB, Van Der Vleuten C, Schuwirth LW, Muijtjens AMM. Broadening perspectives on clinical performance assessment: rethinking the nature of in-training assessment. *Adv Health Sci Educ* 2007; **12**: 239–260.
8. Galbraith RM, Holtman MC, Clyman SG. Use of assessment to reinforce patient safety as a habit. *Qual Saf Health Care* 2006; **15**: i30–i33.
9. Van der Vleuten C. The assessment of professional competence: developments, research and practical implications. *Adv Health Sci Educ* 1996; **(1)**: 41–67.
10. Messick S. Standards of validity and the validity of standards in performance assessment. *Educ Meas: Issues Practice* 1995; **14(4)**: 5–8.
11. Messick S. The interplay of evidence and consequences in the validation of performance assessments. *Educ Res* 1994; **23(2)**: 13–23.
12. Streiner DL, Norman GR. Health measurement scales: a practical guide to their development and use, 2nd edition. Oxford University Press, Oxford, 2001.
13. Downing SM. Validity: on the meaningful interpretation of assessment data. *Med Educ* 2003; **37(9)**: 830–837.

14. Cronbach L, Gleser G, Nanda G, Rajaratnam N. The dependability of behavioural measurements: theory of generalisability for scores and profiles. Wiley, New York, 1972.

15. Cronbach LSRJ. My current thoughts on coefficient alpha and successor procedures. *Educ Psychol Meas* 2004; **64(3)**: 391–418.

16. Norcini JJ, Blank LL, Duffy FD, Fortna GS. The mini-CEX: a method for assessing clinical skills. *Ann Intern Med* 2003; **138(6)**: 476–481.

17. Wilkinson J, Crossley J, Wragg A, Mills P, Cowan G, Wade W. Implementing workplace-based assessment across the medical specialties in the United Kingdom. *Med Educ* 2008; **42**: 364–373.

18. General Medical Council. Good medical practice. GMC, London. www.gmc-uk.org

19. Archer JC, Norcini J, Davies HA. Use of SPRAT for peer review of paediatricians in training. *Br Med J* 2005; **330**: 1251–1253.

20. Archer JC, Norcini J, Southgate L, Heard S, Davies H. Mini-PAT (peer assessment tool): a valid component of a national assessment programme in the UK? *Adv Health Sci Educ* 2006. Published online at http://dx.doi.org/10.1007/s10459-006-9033-3

21. Norman GR. Problem-solving skills, solving problems and problem-based learning. *Med Educ* 1988; **22(4)**: 279–286.

22. Southgate L, Cox J, David T, Hatch D, Howes A, Johnson N *et al.* The General Medical Council's performance procedures: peer review of performance in the workplace. *Med Educ* 2001; **35(Suppl. 1)**: 9–19.

23. Ilgen DR, Barnes-Farrell JL, McKellin DB. Performance appraisal process research in the 1980s: what has it contributed to appraisals in use? *Org Behav Human Decision Proc* 1993; **54**: 321–368.

24. Finn RH. Effects of some variations in rating scale characteristics of the means and reliabilities of ratings. *Educ Psychol Meas* 1972; **32**: 255–265.

25. Lam TC, Klockars AJ. Anchor point effects on the equivalence of questionnaire items. *J Educ Meas* 1982; **19(4)**: 317–322.

26. Miller GA. The magical number seven, plus or minus two: some limits on our capacity for processing information. *Psychol Rev* 1994; **101(2)**: 343–352.

27. Masters JR. The relationship between number of response categories and reliability of Likert-type questionnaires. *J Educ Meas* 1974; **11**: 49–53.

28. Schuwirth LW, Southgate L, Page GG, Paget NS, Lescop JM, Lew SR *et al.* When enough is enough: a conceptual basis for fair and defensible practice performance assessment. *Med Educ* 2002; **36(10)**: 925–930.

29. Jamtvedt G, Young JM, Kristoffersen DT, O'Brien MA, Oxman AD. Audit and feedback: effects on professional practice and health care outcomes. Cochrane Database of Systematic Reviews 2006, Issue 2. Art. No.: CD000259. DOI: 10.1002/14651858. CD000259.pub2.

30. Sargeant JM, Mann K, Sinclair D, Ferrier S, Muirhead P, van der Vleuten C *et al.* Learning in practice: experiences and perceptions of high-scoring physicians. *Acad Med* 2006; **81(7)**: 655–660.

31. Sargeant JM. Understanding the influence of emotions and reflection upon multi-source feedback acceptance and use. In: Sargeant JM (Ed.), Multi-source feedback for physicians learning and change. University of Maastricht, Maastricht, 2006.

32. Kluger AN, DeNisi A. The effects of feedback intervention on performance: a historical review, a meta-analysis, and a preliminary feedback intervention theory. *Psychol Bull* 1996; **119**: 254–284.

33. Holmboe ES, Yepes M, Williams F. Feedback and the mini clinical evaluation exercise. J *Gen Intern Med* 2004; **19**: 558–561.
34. Hewson MG, Little ML. Giving feedback in medical education. Verification of recommended techniques. *J Gen Intern Med* 1998; **13(2)**: 111–116.
35. Ende J, Pomerantz A, Erickson F. Preceptors' strategies for correcting residents in an ambulatory care medicine setting: a qualitative analysis. *Acad Med* 1995; **70**: 224–229.
36. Dudek NL, Marks MB and REgehr G. Failure to fail: the perspectives of clinical supervisors. *Acad Med* 2005; **80(S10)**: S84–S87.
37. Sargeant JM, Mann KV, Ferrier SN, Langille DB, Muirhead PH, Hayes VM *et al.* Responses of rural family physicians and their colleague and co-worker raters to a multi-source feedback process: a pilot study. *Acad Med* 2003; **78**: 42S–44S.
38. Grimshaw J, Eccles M, Tetroe J. Implementing clinical guidelines: current evidence and future implications. *J Cont Educ Health Prof* 2004; **24(Suppl. 1)**: S31–S37.
39. Kruger J and Dunning D. Unskilled and unaware of it: how difficulties in recognising one's own incompetence lead to inflated self-assessments. *J Pers Social Psychol* 1999; **77(6)**: 1121–1134.

Further resources

• Norcini J, Burch V. Workplace-based assessment as an educational tool: AMEE Guide No 31. *Med Teacher* 2007; **29**: 855–871.
• British Medical Association Board of Medical Education. Appraisal: a guide for medical practitioners. BMA, London, 2003. www.bma.org.uk
• www.appraisals.nhs.uk The NHS appraisal toolkit website.

CHAPTER 9

The role of information technology

Sean Smith
The Yorkshire Deanery, University of Leeds, Leeds, UK

Information technology (IT) refers to the use of modern technology, and computers in particular, in the creation, management and use of information. As in all forms of education, and indeed life in general, the use of IT is becoming increasingly prominent in postgraduate medical education. In fact, it is not too difficult to imagine it to be all pervading in the not-too-distant future. While medical training at all stages is essentially hands-on, IT can be used to augment that training and ease the burden of record keeping that comes hand in hand with the Modernising Medical Careers (MMC) agenda.

This chapter introduces some of the most common applications of IT currently employed in postgraduate medical education, in both training and educational contexts, and also attempts to anticipate how aspects of IT may impact on training in the future.

e-learning

IT has been used in education for some time in the form of 'e-learning'. This particular form of learning is becoming increasingly sophisticated and is finding its way into virtually all tertiary education curricula in the UK (Box 9.1).

Box 9.1

The 'e' prefix in e-learning clearly stands for 'electronic'. Few other examples (all of which have appeared in published work recently) are e-moderating, e-assessment, e-portfolios, e-mentoring, e-tutoring, e-citizen, e-commerce, e-book and e-banking.

Essential Guide to Educational Supervision in Postgraduate Medical Education.
Edited by Nicola Cooper and Kirsty Forrest. © 2009 Blackwell Publishing,
ISBN: 978-1-4051-7071-0.

E-learning has developed from the computer-mediated training methods used as long ago as the 1950s and from distance learning methods dating further back than that. Initially the limitations of the technology restricted its use to single computer systems such as a set of terminals in a university computer lab. More recent advances in personal computers combined with simpler development tools have led to a revolution in e-learning. It was inevitable that the growth of the Internet would be exploited for this form of learning.

E-learning may now be regarded as a generic term for a number of modes of learning, for example:

- Web-based learning materials (often embedded in virtual learning environments)
- Online forums/discussion groups
- Online assessments
- Animations
- Real-time chat
- Collaborative software

To complicate things further, there are a number of delivery methods used in the field:

- CD Rom
- DVD
- Web
- Personal digital assistant (PDA)/smart phone.

Given its ubiquitous nature, it is not surprising that the Web has become the most common form of delivery. In fact CDs and/or DVD only tend to be used for media heavy material, when the bandwidth limitations of the Web would impact on download time and frustrate the end user. There are also situations where it may not be convenient to use a PC and content may be developed for the PDA or smart phone in these instances.

There is a wide spectrum of Web-based learning. At the simpler end of the spectrum, tutors may simply make the presentation and word processing files used for slides and handouts available to their students on the Web. This allows easy distribution of a course's support materials and may be supplemented with links to appropriate websites. It is common to translate text and graphics into the Web's native format HTML (hypertext mark-up language). There are many software packages readily available that have fairly sophisticated tools to support this conversion. With some editing, materials can be grouped and structured, making them easier for students to navigate. A desirable enhancement particularly suited to adult learners – as it is believed to encourage a constructivist model of learning – is to link the webpages to online communication tools. Web-based discussion boards/forums are most commonly used, which are technically straightforward but pedagogically (educationally) very rich. Online discussion, tutor support and 'virtual' group work all become possible. If properly planned and supported by the tutor in a role often termed as 'e-moderating', a rich and valuable learning experience may be designed. It is perhaps this aspect of Web-based learning that experts in the field, such as Salmon [1], recognise as being the most educationally valuable. However, it should be noted that this style of teaching requires a significant time commitment from the tutor.

For those with a modicum of technical skill or with good technical support (Box 9.2), it is possible to write interactive simulations and models – this is the next level in our spectrum. Experimenting with even a simple simulation can be a powerful learning experience; however, these applications are often challenging and time-consuming to develop. Somewhat easier to produce, technically at least, are online quizzes. These are often based on multiple-choice questions, multiple response, matching questions or any number of other styles. Such quizzes can be useful for the diagnosis of students' problem areas, learning reinforcement and self-assessment. At the upper end of the Web-materials spectrum are the complex, media-rich, commercial standard materials of full online courses.

Box 9.2

Most universities have a specialist unit dedicated to these simulation methods and other alternative/flexible forms of learning. The titles of these units vary from one institution to the next (e.g. at Leeds University it is the 'Flexible Learning and Development Unit', at Manchester University it is the 'Distributed Learning Team'). Generally they serve to champion e-learning and provide practical help in producing the necessary materials. They should be the first source of advice you seek out if you are considering the development of e-learning materials.

The pros and cons of e-learning

The main advantage of this form of provision (particularly when applied to Web-based learning) is in the unlimited access to the course contents, any time, anywhere. The environment lends itself to flexibility yet at the same time provides permanent access, allowing users to progress at their own pace. This is a particular advantage for shift-workers working within the limitations of the European Working Time Directive. Web-based teaching also offers almost unlimited information resources. In this context, learning should be more creative because students participate actively in selecting information relevant to any given task and in developing knowledge from their own perspective. In contrast to printed media, the use of the Internet allows for the use of more up-to-date information. The learning process can be enhanced using interactive audiovisual elements. From the provider's point of view, the technology allows for economy of scale (in terms of time and finance).

There are, however, disadvantages in delivering courses via the Web. It is important to understand that learning material should be designed with sound educational principles in mind. The learning environment is unstructured and may lead to information overload for the learner. Similarly, without self-discipline, the student may become distracted when navigating through various sources of information. Kroder *et al.* [2] reported that Web-based learning took 20–40% more time and effort on the part of students. In addition, feedback may be delayed as the student does not have immediate interaction with instructors or peers, which may lead to the perception of isolation. It is argued, however, that this can be minimised through the use of communication technology, and that taking the time to reflect on an issue before responding is good educational practice.

In addition to the student-orientated problems that e-learning presents, there are also provider factors. The biggest potential hindrance to the uptake of e-learning is the high initial cost and considerable effort of development. Bacsich and Ash [3] estimated the development time to learning time ratio as between 10:1 and 100:1 depending on the complexity of the learning materials. A second but not insignificant problem may lie with the tutors themselves. The switch to a technology-orientated learning approach requires a significant amount of effort on the part of tutors and can therefore act as a disincentive, particularly for the technophobic.

Horton [4] quotes many instances of studies that have found Web-based learning as effective as traditional methods and a handful of studies demonstrating that Web-based learning was significantly more effective. Similar results were found in a review of e-learning used in continuing medical education in the USA by Wutoh *et al.* [5]. This would suggest that the advantages of the technology outweigh the disadvantages, and that the benefits translate to busy clinicians.

Blended learning

Blended learning seeks to combine the best of both worlds, the flexibility of e-learning methods with the immediacy of face-to-face teaching. We have listed the benefits of e-learning, but that is not to say that traditional methods of teaching do not have their benefits as well. A strict definition of blended learning would be 'the combination of multiple approaches to learning'. However, it is increasingly used to describe programmes that combine technology-based materials and face-to-face sessions. There are many examples of blended learning programmes, the precise composition of which vary greatly. It is essential, however, that each form of learning should complement and integrate with the other and that both clearly satisfy defined learning objectives.

Many postgraduate training programmes are adopting blended learning in response to shorter training times, shift work and an increasing understanding of educational principles. The Radiology Academies are one example. 'Flexible learning for anaesthetic trainees (FLAT)' is another [6].

Potential uses of e-learning in foundation programmes

Higgins *et al.* [7] describe poor attendance of house officers at formal teaching sessions, with a significant number of trainees missing 50% of classes. While this observation described the situation prior to the introduction of MMC, anecdotal evidence would suggest that this state of affairs continues. Various reasons for the poor attendance rates were cited based on responses to anonymous questionnaires completed by junior doctors at the Leicestershire, Northamptonshire and Rutland (LNR) Healthcare Workforce Deanery. Two types of barrier to attendance were identified in the study: 'routine barriers', which related to hospital working patterns, and 'contextual barriers', which referred to the particular hospital post. Routine barriers quoted included on-call work, annual leave, sickness and night shifts, with on-call work being the most commonly reported. Contextual barriers included lack of cover for the post, the ward being too busy, or the house officer's time not being protected effectively. Critically, the doctors' motivation and commitment to the teaching programme were excluded as significant causes of poor attendance.

If we extrapolate the implications of these findings to the wider, national context and accept that the quoted barriers to attendance apply to current foundation programmes, as well as other postgraduate programmes, then we need to consider ways of improving the situation. One such measure may be to introduce the more flexible learning methods offered by e-learning. Indeed the authors suggested the more widespread use of online learning resources to partly alleviate the problem. There are early signs of the adoption of e-learning in foundation training (Box 9.3).

Box 9.3 Web-based module in acute care

Acute care is one of the themes of the foundation programme curriculum. This 'stand alone' module, developed by Leeds clinicians, consists of 10 tutorials that include an introduction with learning objectives and an interactive quiz. Interactivity has been built into the text wherever possible, such as pop-up boxes with either additional information (depending on the context) or an answer to the question just posed. A small number of interactive animations are included as well. The quizzes at the end of each tutorial are designed as informal formative assessments and include a number of question styles from single choice to ordered lists. A running score is displayed but is not ultimately recorded.

(*Continued*)

Box 9.3 (Continued)

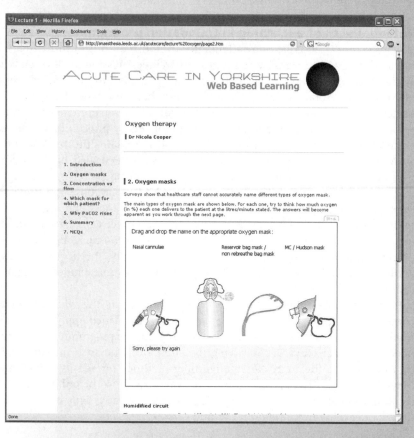

The module was piloted on house officers who had attended an acute care training (ACT) course. Responses to the evaluation that followed completion of the module were very positive, with most participants finding the learning experience a positive one.

Online questionnaires and feedback forms

Questionnaires are particularly useful during periods of change, for example in evaluating the effects afterwards. Feedback forms may also be used as part of the quality assurance process (for details see Chapter 10).

It is now possible to capture this information electronically on the Web. This presents many benefits to both the trainee and the evaluator.

- Greater anonymity for the user
- Availability any time, anywhere
- Instantaneous submission and no need for envelopes or for posting/delivering completed forms

- Assured security if the evaluator chooses to apply password protection to the form
- Data validation to maintain data quality, for example the user forced to submit a date where it is required
- Greater precision of data capture – no handwriting to interpret, no double ticking of boxes
- Seamless data capture – the data can be dropped directly into a database for subsequent analysis without the need for human intervention.

However, Web-based questionnaires lack the immediacy of paper, which can be useful, for example when an evaluation form is being filled in immediately after a training session.

E-portfolios

An integral part of MMC is the portfolio, the now-familiar record of appraisals, assessments, reflection, reviews and evidence of progress. Initially this was a paper-based document but now it is increasingly taking an electronic form.

The concept of e-portfolios is not new. They have been used in education for some time, initially in higher education but increasingly in some schools. An e-portfolio is a compilation of evidence drawn together and maintained by the user, usually on the Web. This can be maintained dynamically over time, which is obviously a key benefit over the paper format. In the general education field, e-portfolios have also been used for personal reflection to evidence educational progress.

At the time of writing, many foundation schools are adopting e-portfolios in preference to the paper version. The e-portfolio has also been adopted

---

Box 9.4

The Yorkshire Deanery has been evaluating the quality of foundation posts using a feedback form for a number of years. Paper forms were used initially. Once the forms were completed they were returned to postgraduate education centre staff, who scanned the forms using Formic supplied software and hardware. The software was then used to capture the submission data and collect it centrally in a database. Data analysis was then undertaken at the end of the year to provide each foundation school and trust with summarised satisfaction scores against set criteria. Comparisons were made between individual trusts and the Deanery as a whole. Longitudinal trends were also presented.

For the last couple of years the Deanery has moved to online forms, which is now the primary means of evaluating foundation posts. Trainees are given a Web address for the form and are asked to complete and submit the form at the end of each post. Data capture and analysis follows the same pattern as before.

(*Continued*)

Box 9.4 (Continued)

Data capture has become far more effective and accurate, manual interpretation of forms is no longer necessary by postgraduate education centre staff and trainees report high satisfaction using the Web-based form. However, removing the postgraduate education centre staff from the feedback process has led to less effective ways of dealing with noncompliance on the part of trainees, and submission rates have fallen slightly.

by several of the Royal Colleges and is finding widespread use in the larger specialties.

The e-portfolio is hosted centrally, but with a username and password the trainees, educational supervisors or administrators may access it from any computer connected to the Internet. The foundation programme e-portfolio currently includes:

- the record of training;
- educational agreements;
- self-assessments;

- personal development plan;
- a reflective log;
- records of appraisals and
- evidence of competence, including work-based assessments and educational supervisor's report.

Why use an e-portfolio rather than a paper-based one? There are several benefits to the electronic version that may explain its growing popularity.

- The e-portfolio is available any time, anywhere.
- Access is specific to the user's role, protecting confidentiality of certain data. For example, the trainees' personal reflections can be restricted to themselves. Notes from review meetings may be restricted to the trainee and his or her educational supervisor.
- Educational supervisors can obtain an overview of review meetings and assessments for all of their trainees. The system will alert the supervisor (via email) of forthcoming meetings or assessments.
- Live evaluation data for trainees (e.g. for 360° feedback) can be viewed and compared to the current national average.

E-induction

Employers are obliged to provide new employees with an induction programme to introduce them to local policies (in particular to health and safety and fire regulations), which presents two problems for junior doctors.

- They may rotate between different hospitals during the course of each year of a programme, and each hospital is likely to have an obligatory induction programme of its own. Potentially, trainees could find themselves attending two to three induction programmes per year.
- To be effective, induction should take place as early as possible in new employment, in other words, just when the trainee is finding his or her feet on a new ward.

E-induction has been seen as a means of overcoming these problems. It is the process of applying e-learning techniques to an induction programme. Essentially, there are two stages to the process. The new employee is presented with information that would otherwise be presented face to face in a lecture (e.g. a fire or handwashing lecture). This electronic presentation is likely to be didactic in nature, but in order for it to be considered as a form of *e-learning* it should include some interactivity so as to engage the learner. This is followed with some form of electronic assessment based on the content presented.

To the employees the assessment serves as a means of ensuring that they have understood and retained the information given, in a formative manner. To the employer it may serve as evidence that the induction programme has been followed, in a summative manner. The assessment(s) are logged to provide evidence that induction has taken place in much the same way that attendance sheets would be kept for a traditional programme. Box 9.5 gives an example.

> **Box 9.5**
>
> The Bradford Teaching Hospitals have adopted a learning management system that allows them to produce an e-induction programme for junior doctors.
>
> New trainees are given a username and password once their employment has been confirmed and before they begin in post. The trainee is then able to log in and view the core online presentations at any time that suits them. Topics include:
> - health and safety;
> - patient safety;
> - fire safety;
> - blood transfusion and
> - infection control.
>
> Following each topic trainees are required to complete a small number of multiple choice questions. They are allowed to complete the questions any number of times but have to pass each element of the programme. The whole programme takes between 1½ and 2 hours to complete.
>
> Scores are tracked by the system. Individuals have a training record that they and their managers can view. The new programme has proved successful, but early experience suggests that following up noncompliance can take a lot of administrator's time.

High-fidelity simulators

Simulation is currently a hot topic in medical education. Simulation can be very basic, for example practicing basic life support on a manikin, or involve high-fidelity simulators – sophisticated computers that aim to make a scenario as realistic as possible. Examples include virtual colonoscopy trainers and SimMan™. Simulation has become more popular because there are a number of barriers to traditional clinical skills learning.
- Learning certain procedures for the first time on patients has become less acceptable.
- Total training time has reduced.
- Some situations (e.g. certain emergencies) are extremely important but rare.
- Regulatory bodies have decreed that certain skills should be assessed.
- Students learn more effectively in a nonthreatening environment.
- There is an emphasis on multidisciplinary team learning.

High-fidelity simulation was addressed by a Best Evidence Medical Education review in 2002 [8], which looked at the factors that make the use of high-fidelity simulators effective from an educational point of view. High-fidelity simulation is increasingly being used in postgraduate medical education, particularly in team training [9].

The future

There are a number of newly emerging technologies that may have some potential application to postgraduate training.

Web 2.0 refers to a significant shift in the use of the Web for collaborative purposes. The term is used particularly for those sites that are characterised by social networking and Web-based communities. User interactivity is the key to Web 2.0, where users can upload as well as download information or browse it. Blogs and wikis are perhaps the two most common manifestations of Web 2.0 at the time of writing.

The term 'blog' is short for 'Web log' and describes a type of online diary or commentary. Blogs are becoming increasingly popular in the education community where they are collectively known as 'edublogs'. They are used by a tutor to provide a commentary on topics currently important to a particular group of students to supplement or reinforce teaching delivered face to face or online. They are particularly useful in a blended learning environment as they maintain the attention and engagement of trainees between face-to-face sessions.

A 'wiki' is a collaborative website that can be directly edited by anyone with access to it (http://en.wikipedia.org/wiki – accessed 04/09/07). It derives from the Hawaiian word for 'fast'. Wikipedia is the most well-known example. A wiki takes the form of a collection of collaborative documents or pages interconnected by hyperlinks. The pages of information are produced and updated by the users themselves. Another essential characteristic of a wiki is the ability to keep a log of the history of a document as it is developed, so the current version can be compared to any previous version. Wikis can be used by a group for educational purposes. For example, a report can be produced collaboratively by a group using a wiki.

References

1. Salmon G. E-moderating: the key to teaching and learning online. Kogan Page, London, 2000.
2. Kroder SL, Suess J, Sachs D. Lessons in launching web based graduate courses. *T.H.E. J* 1998 (May). URL www.thejournal.com/articles/14089
3. Bacsich P, Ash C. Costing the lifecycle of networked learning, documenting the costs from concept to evaluation. *ALT-J* 2000; **8 (1)**: 92–102.
4. Horton WK. Designing web-based training. John Wiley and Sons, New York, 2000.
5. Wutoh R, Boren SA, Balas EA. E-learning: a review of Internet-based continuing medical education. *J Contin Educ Health Prof* 2004; **24**: 20–30.
6. Forrest KA, Smith S, Howell S. A new way of learning – reflections on our first year. Bulletin 28. The Royal College of Anaesthetists, November 2004. URL www.rcoa.ac.uk/docs/Bulletin28.pdf
7. Higgins R, Cavendish S, Gregory R. Class half-empty? Pre-registration house officer attendance at weekly teaching sessions: implications for delivering the new foundation programme curriculum. *Med Educ* 2006; **40**: 877–883.

8. Issenberg SB, McGaghie WC, Petrusa ER, Gordon DL, Scalese RJ. Features and uses of high-fidelity medical simulations that lead to effective learning: a BEME systematic review. *Med Teach* 2005; **27 (2)**: 10–28.

9. The Industrial Psychology Research Centre, Department of Anaesthesia at the University of Aberdeen, and the Scottish Clinical Simulation Centre. Anaesthetists' non-technical skills (ANTS). Also contains a link to the Royal College of Surgeons of Edinburgh and University of Aberdeen project, NOTTS – non-technical skills for surgeons. URL www.abdn.ac.uk/iprc/ants

CHAPTER 10

Quality assurance

Jonathan Beard[1] & Nicola Cooper[2]
[1]University of Sheffield, Sheffield, UK
[2]The Leeds Teaching Hospitals NHS Trust, Leeds, UK

This chapter reviews how the organisations responsible for postgraduate medical education ensure that quality training is being delivered 'on the ground'. Some definitions and the responsibilities of the Postgraduate Medical Education and Training Board (PMETB), deaneries and local education providers are discussed. We then look at what quality assurance (QA) means *in practice* for educational supervisors and training programme directors.

Definitions

Quality assurance is about ensuring that standards are (a) specified and (b) consistently met. It is a concept borrowed from industry, in which a manufacturer guarantees the customer that goods meet the specified standard. In this context, quality can have two meanings:
• The characteristics of a product that satisfy its 'fitness for purpose'.
• A product that conforms to requirements – i.e. is free from defects.
In medical education, 'fitness for purpose' and *standards* are closely related. Standards do not however just focus on the end product, but encompass the nature and organisation of the curriculum, the approaches to teaching and learning (including faculty development) and student assessment. The 'customer' for postgraduate medical education in the UK is the PMETB, which acts on behalf of the Department of Health and the general public.

There is considerable confusion about the difference between quality assurance, quality management and quality control, and many people use these terms interchangeably. The definitions used by the PMETB are as follows:
• *Quality assurance (QA)*
   This encompasses all the policies, standards, systems and processes directed towards ensuring the quality of UK postgraduate medical education.

Essential Guide to Educational Supervision in Postgraduate Medical Education,
1st edition. Edited by Nicola Cooper and Kirsty Forrest. © 2009 Blackwell Publishing,
ISBN: 978-1-4051-7071-0.

- *Quality management (QM)*

  This refers to the arrangements by which the regional postgraduate deaneries discharge their responsibility for the standards and quality of postgraduate medical education. The deaneries work with medical royal
  colleges, faculties and specialist societies, training programme directors,
  trainees and National Health Service (NHS) trusts to ensure that local education and training providers are meeting the PMETB standards.
- *Quality control (QC)*

  This relates to the organisation and processes at local level (e.g. in hospitals and general practices) which are designed to ensure that standards are
  being met.

Quality improvement, yet another term, is implied throughout the whole
quality process. This is the means by which, through critical and continuous
evaluation, standards are continually reviewed and improved.

Organisation

The PMETB is responsible for QA, the deaneries (regional departments of
postgraduate medical education) are responsible for QM and local education
providers (primary and secondary care trusts and their postgraduate medical
education departments) are responsible for QC [1,2].

The PMETB is an independent statutory body, responsible for oversee-
ing and promoting the development of postgraduate medical education and
training for all medical specialties, including general practice, since 2005.
It took over the responsibilities of the Specialist Training Authority of the
Medical Royal Colleges and the Joint Committee on Postgraduate Training
for General Practice. The PMETB's statutory responsibilities include establishing, promoting, developing and maintaining standards and requirements
for postgraduate medical education and training across the UK.

Figure 10.1 illustrates the different levels of QA, QM and QC and how
they relate to each other. The deaneries are responsible for managing the
quality of postgraduate medical education on behalf of the PMETB, and for
maintaining and improving standards over time. The royal colleges, faculties
and specialist societies have an input into the process at all levels.

Quality assurance in postgraduate medical education

Generic standards for training

The PMETB has identified nine domains (areas) in which certain standards
have been set for all medical specialties [3]. These are:

- patient safety;
- QA, review and evaluation;
- equality, diversity and opportunity;
- recruitment, selection and appointment;
- delivery of the curriculum, including assessment;

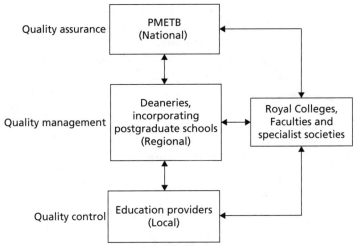

Figure 10.1 The different levels of QA, QM and QC and how they relate to each other.

- support and development of trainees, trainers and local faculty;
- management of education and training;
- educational resources and capacity;
- outcomes.

Within each area, mandatory and developmental (in progress) standards are specified. For example, under 'delivery of the curriculum', one of the mandatory standards is: 'Each programme must show how the posts within it, taken together, will meet the requirements of the curriculum and what must be delivered within each post'.

The quality assurance framework

The PMETB QA framework has five elements (Figure 10.2).

- Standards – standards are set by approving curricula, programmes and posts.
- Shared evidence – evidence such as survey data, reports, number of trainees by specialty are shared.
- Surveys – deaneries, trainers and trainees are surveyed.
- Visits to deaneries – deaneries are visited to scrutinise their QM by sampling specialties.
- Response to concerns – concerns from PMETB findings, external bodies, for example colleges, trainers or trainees, are studied.

The PMETB also operates a system of triggered visits. Triggered visits are undertaken where there may be a serious educational failure that requires rapid investigation and where concerns cannot be dealt with in any other way. They are arranged by the PMETB in partnership with the relevant medical royal college and deanery.

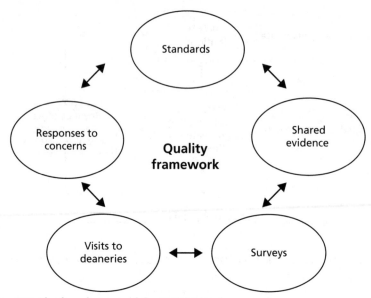

Figure 10.2 The five elements of the PMETB QA framework.

The QA framework is similar to an audit cycle – both aim to measure out-comes against defined criteria, with a view to continually improving standards.

It could be argued that it is the deaneries, not the PMETB, who should be responsible for assessing the quality of postgraduate medical education because this is a QM function. The PMETB should focus on ensuring that QM and QC systems are in place and operational, because this is their QA function. However, the PMETB would argue that it cannot legally delegate its powers of approval and it needs to verify the evidence it receives. This is its reason for sampling specialities during deanery visits. The purpose of such sampling is to verify the deanery's QM and QC processes, not to specifically check on the chosen specialities.

Quality management

QM is a process that operates at a regional level (e.g. throughout Yorkshire). Most deaneries have instituted a QM process that reviews the quality of education provided by each hospital and primary care trust in their area on an annual basis, as part of their educational contract with that provider. The results of trainee questionnaires, the annual report from the director of postgraduate medical education and any issues arising from external visits are discussed with the relevant chief executive, medical director, director of postgraduate medical education and specialty leads.

In saying 'the deanery' is responsible for QM, we mean deanery staff, regional college appointees, heads of postgraduate schools and specialty training committee chairmen. All of these people are responsible for the QM process within their respective spheres.

Quality control

The responsibility for day-to-day QC lies with the director of postgraduate medical education, who is usually appointed jointly by a trust and its deanery. This function is, in turn, delegated to foundation or specialty programme directors, supported by the trust's postgraduate medical education centre staff.

Local education providers are directly responsible for six out of the nine areas in the PMETB generic standards for training: patient safety; equality, diversity and opportunity (which relates to flexible training and disabilities); delivery of the curriculum; support of trainees, trainers and local faculty; management of education and training; educational resources and capacity.

But what does this mean *in practice* for training programme directors and educational supervisors?

Quality control in practice

On a personal level, most educational supervisors want to do their job well. They will read about the subject, attend courses, talk to colleagues and think about their role as an educational supervisor. However, educational supervisors and training programme directors sometimes fall short when it comes to QC and the bigger picture.

Think about the following main local activities that are linked to the PMETB generic standards for training listed in the preceding text:
- induction;
- maintenance of appropriate clinical supervision, duties and rotas;
- delivery of the curriculum;
- educational supervisor development and support;
- mechanisms to identify and deal with problems.

Quality control is about ensuring that these things are in place. But it is more than that – it is about whether or not they are also 'fit for purpose'. This links in with the idea of *quality improvement*. Pause for a moment to ask yourself the following questions about your own situation:
- Is there an adequate induction programme for all new trainees?
- Has the training programme been designed with the curriculum in mind?
- How do we evaluate our training programmes?
- Are all educational supervisors trained in the curriculum, portfolio, assessments, appraisal and counselling skills, and in giving feedback and careers advice?
- How are problem trainees and trainers managed?
- Do we routinely use exit questionnaires?
- What evidence can we provide that our local activities meet the required standards?

You may know the answers to many of these questions, but may have spotted gaps in the QC process in your own institution. Gathering information pertaining to the PMETB standards and providing evidence of QC is a form of evaluation.

Evaluation

Quality control involves institutional self-evaluation. Formal evaluation (as opposed to informal) is accessible and used to provide evidence for the QA process. It is also used for quality improvement. Evaluation involves an appraisal of:

- intentions (the curriculum);
- outcomes (trainee performance);
- processes (the programme organisation and teaching–learning in action).

All three are necessary and complementary. However, it is common to find that only the first two are formally evaluated as part of QC in postgraduate medical education, leaving out the important aspect of processes. In other words, we tend to tick a box that something has been done, and give very little consideration as to whether or not it was educationally effective. As an editorial in the BMJ about foundation programmes articulated, 'High quality teaching and learning do not happen by accident: a curriculum is initially no more than a document' [4].

An appraisal of outcomes alone could lead to the wrong conclusions. For example, trainee performance could be measured using the pass rate for royal college examinations. However, knowing that all the local trainees attend an expensive crammer course at the other end of the country prior to their examinations might question the educational effectiveness of a local training programme.

Box 10.1 illustrates a simple example of evaluation in action.

Box 10.1 Evaluation in action

A consultant was asked to organise a new training programme for specialty registrars in a particular hospital. Four new posts were to be converted from old senior house officer posts in various subspecialties. At a superficial level, all that was required was to organise their timetables and meet them on the first day. However, consideration of the different aspects of *quality control* revealed several other areas that needed to be addressed.

These included:
- induction;
- maintenance of appropriate clinical supervision, duties and rotas;
- delivery of the curriculum, which included teaching and learning methods;

(Continued)

Box 10.1 (Continued)

- educational supervisor development and support;
- mechanisms to deal with problems.

Once the programme was running, formal evaluation would be required to appraise the intentions, outcomes and processes of all of the above, as part of an ongoing *quality improvement* programme.

This seemed like a lot of work, so the following simple questions were asked to get the process started:

- Does everyone involved know what the intentions are?
- Is everyone involved performing satisfactorily against the standards set?
- Are the processes clear?
- Are the processes effective?
- Is everyone involved – trainers and trainees – equipped for their role?

Questionnaires, surveys or checklists could be used to document the answers to these questions.

As an exercise, imagine your own situation, or that you have been asked to run this new training programme. Once the evaluation is done, you might need to think in terms of quality improvement: are there better ways of communicating intentions, making the programme more educationally effective, or ensuring that educational supervisors and trainees are equipped for their role? An evaluation might throw up several different issues and there are many different ways in which to approach them.

Quality improvement

Quality improvement occurs *as a result of* institutional evaluation. As the PMETB QA framework is similar to an audit cycle, quality improvement is a key part of the process. But feedback alone after an evaluation does not tend to result in real change. Multifactorial interventions are more likely to be successful, and thinking in terms of the following categories can be useful [5]:

- barriers;
- education and training;
- systems;
- physical facilities;
- staffing;
- the involvement of the entire clinical team, including management.

A more in-depth approach to evaluation and quality improvement can result in educationally effective re-design of postgraduate training programmes [6].

Educational supervisor development and support

One aspect of QC on which we will focus is educational supervisor development and support. There is a consensus among responsible bodies, educational literature, trainees and educational supervisors themselves that educational supervisors should have training in the relevant curriculum, portfolio, assessments, appraisal and counselling skills, and in giving feedback and careers advice. As the PMETB puts it: 'Educational supervisors in hospital and community settings must have been trained and selected for the role. Resources and time must be available for this task to be carried out and included in their job and personal development plans' [3].

The responsibility for ensuring that this happens lies with the director of postgraduate medical education in a trust, and as mentioned before, is delegated to foundation or specialty programme directors, supported by the trust's postgraduate medical education centre staff. But the deanery works with trusts to ensure standards as well. One of the ways it does this is by providing a range of courses on employment and educational supervisory topics. The royal colleges also run regular courses on specialty topics such as their curriculum, assessment process and portfolios.

Faculty development interventions result in positive changes in the knowledge, skills and attitudes of educational supervisors. However, key features of effective development are experiential learning, feedback and effective peer relationships, in addition to educationally well-designed courses [7].

Workplace-based assessment (WBA) is now commonplace in postgraduate medical education. Although assessments vary slightly depending on the programme, the common ones in use are:
- mini-CEX (clinical evaluation exercise);
- DOPS (direct observation of procedural skills);
- 360° feedback;
- CbD (case-based discussion).

These are discussed further in Chapter 8. The reliability of WBA is improved through regular use, multiple assessors and training in objective assessment and giving feedback [8]. It therefore makes sense for all senior clinicians (including specialty registrars and some nonmedical staff) to be trained in WBA. It is often more feasible for training to be organised on a trust basis by the director of postgraduate medical education, as the foundation and most specialty programmes incorporate WBA in their competency-based curricula. One way to organise such training is through regular lunchtime workshops in the local postgraduate medical education centre.

Educational supervisors need additional training in the relevant curriculum, portfolio and appraisal process. This is best delivered through deanery, faculty or college courses. The National Association of Clinical Tutors runs regular workshops that cover these topics [9]. All educational supervisors should be allocated enough time in their job plan to perform their role. About one hour per week per trainee is recommended. This is usually achieved through the annual job planning process and may require the involvement of the director of postgraduate medical education.

Conclusions – the role of the educational supervisor

Having outlined the 'big picture' when it comes to QA, it can be said that educational supervisors themselves have a professional responsibility to ensure they get the training they need to play their part in delivering the PMETB generic standards for training. The General Medical Council document *The Doctor as Teacher* [10] lists the personal attributes of a doctor with responsibilities for educational supervision. These attributes include:

- enthusiasm for his or her specialty;
- a personal commitment to teaching and learning;
- an understanding of the principles of education as applied to medicine;
- a willingness to develop both as a doctor and as a teacher;
- a commitment to audit and peer review of his or her teaching.

From this list it is clear that enthusiasm, a commitment to personal development and a willingness to develop as an educator are attributes of a good educational supervisor. These personal attributes are a key ingredient in the overall recipe for QA, and should lead to educational supervisors actively seeking the training and resources they need.

References

1. The PMETB Quality Framework for postgraduate medical education and training in the UK. PMETB, London, 2007. Available at www.pmetb.org.uk
2. PMETB. Operational Guide for the PMETB Quality Framework. PMETB, London, 2007. Available at www.pmetb.org.uk
3. PMETB. Generic standards for training. PMETB, London, 2007. Available at www.pmetb.org.uk
4. Hays R. Foundation Programme for newly qualified doctors. *Br Med J* 2005; **331**: 465–466.
5. Cooper N, Forrest K, Cramp P. Audit. In: Essential guide to generic skills. Blackwell/BMJ, Oxford, 2006.
6. Duffy S, Jha V, Kaufmann S. The Yorkshire Modular Training Programme: a model for structured training and quality assurance in obstetrics and gynaecology. *Med Teacher* 2004; **26 (6)**: 540–544.
7. Steinert Y, Mann K, Centeno A *et al.* A systematic review of faculty development initiatives designed to improve teaching effectiveness in medical education. BEME (best evidence in medical education) Guide No 8. *Med Teacher* 2006; **28 (6)**: 497–526.
8. Beard JD, Bussey M. Workplace-based assessment. *Ann R Coll Surg Engl (Suppl)* 2007; **89**: 158–160.
9. www.nact.org.uk The National Association of Clinical Tutors website.
10. General Medical Council. The doctor as teacher. GMC, London, 1999.

Further resources

- Ramani S. Twelve tips to promote excellence in medical teaching. Medical Teacher 2006; **28(1)**: 19–23.
- Mclean M, Cilliers F, Van Wyk JM. Faculty development: yesterday, today and tomorrow. AMEE guide no 36. Medical Teacher 2008; 30: 555–84.

Appendix 1

The following section has been contributed by Judy McKimm and Rosalind Roden. They have supplied scenarios to accompany their chapters. There is an obvious overlap between personal support, mentoring and dealing with doctors in difficulty, which the following scenarios illustrate perfectly. Both authors have a vast knowledge of these situations and the scenarios below reflect the most common situations that arise. The scenarios are not meant to give definitive answers to the questions raised, rather to provide a framework within which to act if you are presented with a similar situation.

Chapter 2 – Personal support and mentoring
Judy McKimm

Each of the following case scenarios is linked to a section in Chapter 2. They are meant as triggers for thinking about some of the issues discussed and are written from different standpoints. There is no separate discussion section here; readers are advised to refer back to the chapter.

What is personal support?

You are the educational supervisor for a new foundation programme trainee. The trainee is a very bright young man, is very keen to do a good job and is extremely enthusiastic. At the first meeting he asks you for a time each week when he can meet with you to discuss progress. When you point out that your meetings with him will be less frequent than this, he tells you that he is dyslexic, has received support throughout his undergraduate course and was led to believe that this would continue with special support in the foundation years.

What do you say to the trainee at the meeting and what are your next steps after the meeting?

Principles underpinning personal support
At the first meeting with your supervisee you start to set out your ground rules in the form of a 'learning contract'. The supervisee says that he or she does not see the need for this – 'everyone else' does things more informally and this has always worked in the past.

Essential Guide to Educational Supervision in Postgraduate Medical Education.
Edited by Nicola Cooper MRCP. copyright symbol Year Blackwell Publishing, ISBN: 978-1-4051-7071-0.

What do you say to the supervisee, how would you explain the importance of ground rules and contracts and what are the core elements of the learning contract that you would want to see in place at this first meeting?

Role boundaries

Your trainee has struggled through his assessments, barely passing each of them and receiving poor feedback from most assessors. You set up a meeting with him to discuss the issues and identify a strategy.

What do you think are the key roles that you need to take on to help the trainee and who else can you contact to help support the trainee achieve his educational objectives?

Providing support through change and transition

Your foundation programme trainee telephones you in tears. She tells you that she has been working with one of the registrars who has told her that 'everything' she is doing is substandard and that the registrar even wonders why she ever thought of practicing medicine. You have also had some informal feedback from others working with your trainee, which suggests she is not gearing up to the demands of the job as well as she might.

How might you structure a conversation with your trainee using the 'competence curve'?

Structuring meetings

Your trainee meets with you regularly and is always very forthcoming and insightful about all aspects of her training. However, you feel that you know nothing of her life outside work and that you do not really know her as a person. No one has flagged up any issues about her work or assessments.

What, if anything, could or should you do in terms of providing additional personal support to this trainee?

Personal support and confidentiality

At a regular meeting with your registrar, he tells you that he wants to share something with you and ask for your advice. He says that he is finally able to admit to himself and accept that he is gay. He is planning to 'come out' to colleagues, family and friends. He adds that although he is sure of his sexuality he is very worried about the implications for his career and asks if you think he should 'stay in the closet'.

What might you say to your registrar? What issues might you have to consider in relation to confidentiality and your own feelings and position?

Self-care

A colleague who is also an educational supervisor chats with you over coffee and tells you that he has been supervising a trainee for a month during which time the trainee has had some personal difficulties. Your colleague has spent a lot of time with the trainee, providing a lot of personal support. Your colleague says that he feels he is doing a great job, and that he is seeing the trainee every evening over a drink to help her and give her a little more support.

What would you say to your colleague? And what might you do if the situation continued?

Mentoring

You are a consultant in acute medicine and have been asked by a younger consultant colleague if you will be his mentor.

What are some of the questions that you might want to ask of your colleague before you begin and what are some of the principles that you would want to have agreed before you act as a mentor?

Power

You are an experienced educational supervisor and consultant in general surgery whose current trainee is a Muslim woman. At each meeting you find that all your suggestions are agreed with, and that your trainee is very diffident. You suspect that she is intimidated by you or your position and that it might also be based on your race/ethnic background.

How might you address this with the trainee? What exactly might you say? And what other alternatives might be open to you?

Chapter 3 – Doctors in difficulty
Rosalind Roden

The following case histories are written to accompany Chapter 3. Each of these case histories is written from a different standpoint. Imagine what you would do in that situation before looking at some suggested points of action in the discussion section that follows.

Case 1

You are the educational supervisor for a foundation programme trainee. You are currently also the clinical supervisor. It is 4 weeks into the placement and the doctor is visibly struggling. There have been several occasions when he has demonstrated poor clinical knowledge and practical skills. His time-keeping is not good and the nurses report breakdowns in communication. You have reviewed his clinical notes and have also noticed that his standard of documentation and note-keeping is poor.

Case 2

You are a consultant in acute medicine. You are worried about one of your registrars. There have been no previous concerns. You have noticed in the last 6 weeks that she seems to lack concentration, and on a number of occasions has turned up late for work or phoned in sick at short notice. You have also noted that she has failed to progress recently with her research project which she had previously been enthusiastic about. At a recent case presentation she appeared unprepared and could not answer questions.

You arranged to speak to the trainee who immediately breaks down in tears and explains that her single surviving parent has been diagnosed with cancer. The trainee has moved in as her parent's carer and is commuting a distance to work and struggling to cope. She is very concerned about her career. She is aware that she is not performing as she should but feels she has a responsibility and a duty to look after her sick parent.

Case 3

You are a consultant in general surgery. During an appraisal the trainee announces unexpectedly that he is considering a career change. He has become increasingly disillusioned with surgery and is considering a move to general practice or a move away from medicine entirely. He states that he does not need to discuss it further, as he has already discussed this with friends and feels that the move is inevitable.

Case 4

You are a consultant in anaesthesia. One of your trainees has been off for 12 months receiving treatment for lymphoma. She has done extremely well and is now in remission. She comes to see you to ask if she can return to work the following week. She says she feels she has been off work long enough and would like to get right back in and take part in the on-call rota. She seems cheerful and positive in her approach.

Case 5

You are a staff grade in emergency medicine. You are on a late shift with a foundation doctor. Over a cup of coffee the foundation doctor tells you that he is becoming increasingly unhappy in the job and is thinking of resigning. Some gentle exploring of the situation reveals that the doctor is feeling bullied and intimidated by one of the specialty trainees. The doctor says that he is constantly being told off, often in front of patients or other staff and on one occasion the specialty trainee has told him that he is 'useless'.

Case 6

You are a consultant in paediatrics. You receive a letter from a doctor who worked with you 5 years ago as senior house officer. You were aware that some time after leaving your department the doctor was convicted of a criminal act and was suspended for a period of time. You have not heard from the doctor since. The doctor writes in the letter that he has now been successfully rehabilitated. He has recently attended a fitness to practice panel at the General Medical Council. His undertakings have been lifted and he has been told that he should seek advice from local sources as to a potential pathway to return to work. The doctor does not know what to do next. He asks for your advice regarding a clinical attachment. He states he always found you helpful in the past and feels he cannot approach anyone else.

Case 7

A close colleague is going through a difficult time at home. You are aware that his marriage is breaking up. You become increasingly concerned about your colleague's appearance at work. He frequently appears late for clinics and leaves early. Your colleague begins to look dishevelled and untidy. On several occasions you notice the smell of stale alcohol on his breath. When he is at work, you observe that his performance is good and you have had no major concerns voiced to you by other members of staff. However someone else has commented that the doctor 'seems to have lost his iron and his alarm clock'.

Discussion

Case 1

A problem has clearly been identified and needs to be discussed and action taken. As much information as possible should be gathered. Information obtained from other sources such as the nursing staff should be clearly documented and dated. An example of the doctor's clinical records may be helpful. Once you feel you have adequate objective information you should arrange to see the trainee for a meeting. Ways of introducing the issue are outlined in Box 3.4. Explain to the doctor that you are concerned about his performance. Listen to his side of the story. First try to provide objective evidence that there is a problem.

If the problems identified appear to be of a relatively minor nature, then it may be possible to resolve them by a discussion between the educational supervisor and the trainee. This should take the form of setting goals and standards that must be achieved within a set time. In most cases, however, it would be appropriate to inform the foundation programme director that such a discussion has taken place and action put in place to resolve the problems. If the performance problems are of a more serious nature, then further action may be needed. If it is felt that patients are potentially at risk then it may be necessary to place the trainee in a fully supervised post. This might preclude the trainee taking part in out-of-hours work. Such an action will inevitably involve the foundation programme director and possibly the postgraduate dean. As before, clear goals, standards and time frames must be established prior to the doctor being placed on a period of supervised training.

The trainee's portfolio should also be carefully reviewed. This may highlight that there have been issues in previous posts that should have been communicated. Particular note should be made as to whether the doctor is achieving progress in terms of his assessments. The doctor should be carefully monitored throughout the remainder of his training programme.

Case 2

This is an example of a doctor who has been performing well but then has a critical personal event occurring in her life that affects her work situation. The important thing is to realise that this is the issue and then see what can be done to help. The doctor has already realised that she is underperforming and this is obviously adding to her concerns.

Initially a short period of leave or carer's leave could be arranged. This will allow the doctor to establish some domestic arrangements and perhaps resource some external help. If the doctor wishes to go on caring for her parent herself in the medium to long term then advice should be sought from the deanery. It is possible that funds may be available from the less than full-time training budget to allow the doctor some time to look after her parent without abandoning her career. Alternatively, it may be possible to modify the rota for a period of time such that the doctor's hours are more compatible with being able to look after her parent.

The training programme director should be involved, although it is likely that most arrangements can be made between the educational supervisor, the trainee and the deanery. If the doctor requires a prolonged period of absence from work then it may be possible to arrange a career break with a suitable 'keep in touch' mechanism. The fact that the doctor wishes to care for her relative during this difficult time should be supported and applauded, not regarded as a failure in performance.

Case 3

Most doctors at some point during their career have doubts about whether or not they are in the right specialty or job. Many take this no further than discussing it with friends or families, some will discuss it with educational supervisors and others will actually move to a new specialty or career. The important thing is that these are enlightened discussions and the individual has the opportunity to explore all possibilities and in particular the reasons for leaving his or her current post.

First engage the trainee and explain that you would like to help him make these difficult career choices. Discussions should take place between yourself and the trainee as to why he is not enjoying the specialty and what he seeks in a career change. Is there anything that can be done to improve his current dissatisfaction with the job? Given that the doctor is already established in surgical training, it would also be appropriate to consider involving the deanery. It is likely that it will have a careers advisor who will also be able to help, particularly if the doctor wishes to explore other possible specialties.

In a situation when a doctor is considering a significant career change, it is essential that he fully explores the reasons for this and the likely changes this is going to have on the way he works. Some doctors regard general practice as a 'way out' of difficult career situations and it is extremely important that doctors are counselled as to what this career involves and what skills and attributes are essential in order to be a good general practitioner. See Chapter 4 for further resources in seeking a career outside medicine.

Case 4

After a prolonged period of sickness (particularly in which the doctor has been through a physical and emotional turmoil) a supported return to work is essential. It is possible that the doctor has already been seen by the occupational health department, but if not, she should be referred. A consultant in occupational health will be able to give advice as to when the doctor should return to work and how a graded return can be arranged. The training programme director should also be informed.

The doctor should start with daytime work initially. This should be less than full time and the doctor should gradually build up to a full daytime working week before considering out-of-hours work. The speed of return will depend very much on the level the trainee was at when she became sick and on her own personal skills and attributes. The educational supervisor will need to be involved closely.

In an acute specialty such as anaesthesia, or where the absence has been prolonged, it may be necessary to have a period of supervised work at the start of the graded return. It may also be advisable that the doctor is reassessed on core competencies, particularly if she has been out of an acute specialty for more than a few months.

Case 5

Bullying is an extremely serious allegation that cannot be ignored. It is clear that this doctor feels upset and frightened as he is considering resigning from his post. The situation is difficult because the alleged perpetrator is a colleague of yours. You must explain to the foundation doctor that this needs to be discussed with more senior colleagues and that he should not resign from his post at this stage.

The next day you should speak confidentially with your consultant. It would be helpful to have documented what the foundation doctor said and your own response. It is the duty of your consultant to explore the situation further. This will involve speaking to all parties and taking statements from both the doctors involved. It is important not to move quickly to blaming anybody. There are always two sides to every story and there are doctors who have been accused of bullying but were subsequently found to have behaved in a professional and reasonable manner – their actions were misinterpreted or misconstrued. The important thing is that once the allegation has been made it cannot be ignored.

Case 6

Returning to a career in medicine following a suspension and reinstatement is an extremely difficult and challenging pathway. It is likely that your local deanery will have had previous experience of dealing with similar situations. Encourage the doctor to approach the deanery and there will need to be correspondence between the deanery and the medical advisors at the GMC. The exact nature of the doctor's situation should be established. A return to ad hoc locum work is generally not advised or permitted by the GMC.

After a period of absence from clinical work the doctor will require retraining. There may be deanery resources to facilitate this. The medical director of the trust in which the doctor is placed must be fully aware of the situation and the doctor can only return to unsupervised clinical work with the expressed permission of the GMC.

The important issue here is to make sure the doctor has contact with the appropriate resources. While it would be unwise to paint an unrealistic picture of the return to work process, it is also essential to give the doctor support and encouragement during this time. While the process should be managed by the deanery, there is no reason why you should not help the doctor as a mentor, particularly if he has worked with you previously and you have a good knowledge of his clinical abilities. You are not in a position to offer this doctor a clinical attachment without further formal discussions with the GMC, the deanery and the trust.

Case 7

It can be extremely difficult to support a colleague during a domestic crisis unless he asks for help. Enquiries of concern may be regarded as interfering or potentially casting doubts on the doctor's clinical performance. In this situation the doctor's appearance has changed and his time-keeping is suffering. Otherwise he is performing as normal. Outward appearances are not everything, but a sudden change in style could be a cause for concern. Poor time-keeping will inevitably cause problems in the workplace. The suggestion that the doctor may be drinking excessively after work is a concern on the background of his marriage break-up.

It should be possible to approach the situation in a sympathetic and supportive way. Arranging to have a cup of coffee or tea together at the end of a clinic may give you the opportunity to gently explain that you are worried about his well-being. It is quite possible that if the doctor is consumed with problems at home, he will not have noticed that this is having an effect on his appearance at work. It may come as quite a shock to him and you may need to be supportive once you have voiced your concerns. You should emphasise that this is a personal approach and nobody else has expressed concerns about his performance. In particular, say that you have no worries about his clinical work. It may be best at this early stage not to dwell on the slightly poor time-keeping. Similarly, it may be better to wait until a rapport has been established before asking whether there are issues regarding alcohol intake.

The British Medical Association's confidential counselling service may be able to help this doctor through a difficult time. Sometimes a short period of annual leave is helpful in order to address work–life balance issues. Often just being aware that a colleague is concerned and is there to talk to is sufficient. If your colleague's behaviour continues to cause you concern then you may need to take further action. First you should try talking to your colleague again. Encourage him to seek help and particularly to talk to his own general practitioner if he is feeling under stress at work and home. Explain that you are still very concerned about him.

If your colleague still does not seem to be responding to your advice and you continue to have concerns, then the time has come to share these with someone else. A more senior colleague is probably the most appropriate person to speak to, or the clinical head of your department. Sometimes people fail to respond to a single opinion, but when this is backed up by someone else, they realise there is a problem.

Further help might involve a temporary adjustment in his job plan and further encouragement to seek help from a counsellor or mentor. Situations like this are not uncommon. Most people will get through difficult times in their lives with support and understanding from colleagues.

Appendix 2

Alastair McGowan
NHS Education for Scotland, Glasgow, UK

The following is a brief history of the development of foundation programmes and the current proposed postgraduate medical training structure in the UK.

While this information does not have a direct impact on how to be an educational supervisor, it does provide some useful information about the history and current training structure.

History of the foundation programmes

At the time of the inception of the National Health Service in 1948, the undergraduate curriculum was designed to produce a doctor who would be safe to enter unsupervised practice at the time of qualification. In 1950, the Royal College of Physicians of London and the General Medical Council (GMC) agreed that it was no longer possible to achieve this.

The Medical Act of that year established that from 1st January 1953, full registration would not be granted without proof of postqualification experience [1,2]. From that time, newly qualified doctors have been required to work as preregistration house officers (PRHO) at an approved hospital or other institution for 12 months before being fully registered.

Generally the PRHO year was successfully completed simply by finishing it.

Provided performance was deemed adequate – usually by the lack of any specific comment otherwise – a certificate of satisfactory service would be issued by the training hospital for each post. At the end of this period of general clinical training, the doctor could be fully registered with the GMC and was free, in theory, to start practice anywhere. In reality, those who continued in hospital training were still working under supervision and most, but not all of those who entered general practice, found posts as an assistant in the first instance [3].

The PRHO year has continued under the remit of the GMC with some modifications that have allowed a more broad-based experience, most notably in general practice.

Quality assurance is delegated by the GMC to medical schools, and commonly from the medical schools to postgraduate deaneries. Over time, there

Essential Guide to Educational Supervision in Postgraduate Medical Education, 1st edition. Edited by Nicola Cooper and Kirsty Forrest. © 2009 Blackwell Publishing, ISBN: 978-1-4051-7071-0.

has been a steady progression of guidance and structure in the form of the GMC document, 'The New Doctor', the establishment of educational supervisors, and more formal processes of appraisal and assessment that have strengthened the learning experience during general clinical training.

The origins of foundation programmes

In the Chief Medical Officer's report, 'Unfinished Business' in 2002, a new career structure in postgraduate medicine was proposed. This built on the work by the previous Chief Medical Officer, Sir Kenneth Calman, which reformed specialist training and merged the old registrar and senior registrar grades. These proposals were taken forward under the banner 'Modernising Medical Careers (MMC)' by the four UK health ministers.

'Unfinished Business' contains the first description of the foundation programme:

> Following graduation, all doctors will enter first a two year foundation programme which includes the current preregistration year. An objective of the foundation programme would be to develop and enhance core or generic clinical skills essential for all doctors (e.g. team-working, communication, ability to produce high standards of clinical governance and patient safety, expertise in accessing, appraising and using evidence as well as time management skills). [4]

This broad outline was further developed by a working group and then a committee of the Academy of Medical Royal Colleges to produce the 'Curriculum for the Foundation Years in Postgraduate Education and Training' in 2005. An operational framework for foundation training was developed by the MMC team and published in the same year.

A central principle of MMC and a central theme of the foundation curriculum is that 'doctors are specifically trained early in their careers to provide safe patient care and to be confident in their management of acutely ill patients'. Many of the competencies and assessments in the foundation curriculum are orientated around this requirement.

The Academy's foundation programme committee debated several times whether or not the second foundation year should be 'themed', that is undertaken within the chosen career specialty of the trainee. Such an arrangement would have the advantage that competencies gained in the first year could be further developed and contextualised within the setting of the trainee's career choice. The consensus view at that time, however, was that given both trainers' and trainees' lack of familiarity with the foundation curriculum, there was a substantial risk that both would pay less attention to it than to the specialty curriculum and so some of its aims would be diluted.

One of the major innovations of foundation programmes has been the embedding of workplace-based assessments (WBA) within the curriculum. In the context of the foundation programme, the development of these tools was undertaken by a group originally established by the London Deanery but thereafter aligned to and with membership from the Academy's foundation programme committee. Development of the assessment tools was followed by widespread assessor training. The role of WBA within the curriculum has resulted in these tools now being in widespread use.

Such is the face validity of WBAs that they, or variations of them, are currently listed on virtually every college website as part of their assessment package for specialty training – and potentially for continuing professional development as well. Formal work to establish a more robust evidence-base for the use of WBAs in postgraduate medical curricula is being undertaken by various agencies including the Academy of Medical Royal Colleges.

The future of foundation programmes

After the problematic recruitment round of 2007, an independent inquiry into MMC was established. Its findings (the Tooke report: 'Aspiring to Excellence') were published in 2008 [5]. The interim report received a substantial level of agreement with 87% of respondents supporting its recommendations and only 4% disagreeing.

One of the main issues of contention, however, was the inquiry's recommendation to uncouple the two foundation years and to move the second year to become part of a three-year 'core training' block. This move would

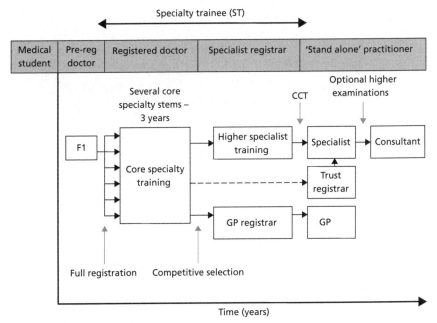

F1 = Foundation 1 (house officer)
GP = General Practitioner
CCT = Certificate of Completion of Training

Figure A2.1 Proposed structure for postgraduate medical training.

effectively introduce the 'themed' Foundation year 2 which was an option considered at the inception of the programme.

Tooke's last comment on this subject forms an appropriate end to this short history of foundation programmes: 'The valuable elements and integrity of the current two-year foundation curriculum should be maintained with a move to "themed" core year 1' [5].

The current proposed structure for postgraduate medical training is shown in Figure A2.1.

References

1. Leading article. Women in medicine. *Br Med J* 1950; **2**: 822.
2. Irvine D. A short history of the General Medical Council. *Med Educ* 2006; **40**: 202–211.
3. Rivett G. From the cradle to the grave: 50 years of the NHS. Kings Fund, London, 1998.
4. Sir Liam Donaldson. Unfinished business: proposals for reform of the senior house officer grade. Department of Health, London, 2002.
5. Tooke J, Ashtiany S, Carter D *et al*. Aspiring to excellence: final report of the independent inquiry into Modernising Medical Careers. www.mmcinquiry.co.uk 2008.

Index